STARLiTE
The Secret Lomi

Discovering the sacred touch of aloha

KEVIN ENGLAND D.C.,D.D.

STARLiTE - The Secret Lomi
Discovering the sacred touch of aloha

First published in 2013 by
Panoma Press Ltd
48 St Vincent Drive, St Albans, Herts, AL1 5SJ UK

info@panomapress.com
www.panomapress.com

Cover design by Michael Inns
Artwork by Karen Gladwell

Printed on acid-free paper from managed forests. This book is printed on demand to fulfill orders, so no copies will be remaindered or pulped.

ISBN 978-1-909623-14-9

Contents

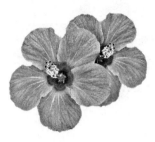

About the author

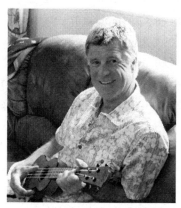

Kevin England D.C., D.D.

Kevin has spent over 40 years practicing the healing arts. He was first introduced to Swedish massage at a time when it was considered 'very new age', something that was 'way out there' and practiced only by hippies on pot. 1968 was the age of Aquarius and an awakening of consciousness for a whole new generation, a time that led to a new spiritual paradigm. While still at school, he suffered a serious knee injury (there was no keyhole surgery in those days) that put paid to a promising sports career, but as one door closed another opened. What followed was six months of intensive injury rehabilitation and an introduction to the healing arts by a blind, retired physiotherapist from Sweden, who became a friend and mentor. Lisbet shared her knowledge of physical therapy, Swedish massage and her love for the joy of life; in return Kevin would collect her shopping and do odd jobs around her home. This friendship of a teenage boy and a 78 year-old 'free spirit' was to have a lifelong effect on him; they shared many happy hours together before she passed away two years later.

Over the last half century, Kevin has worked at the cutting edge of complementary therapy. In the 1970s, armed with a First Aid certificate, and massage and injury rehab knowledge, he worked with local soccer clubs as a sports therapist long before the term was even invented. He studied soft tissue manipulation and osteopathic techniques at Westminster University under the tutelage of the great Leon Chaitow and physiotherapy with the SMAE Institute in London. He completed the Football Association's Diploma course in Sports Injury Management at the National Sports Medicine Centre at Lillishall. In 1998 he graduated from the McTimoney Chiropractic College in Oxford, spent a couple of years as a techniques instructor at the College, and as a postgraduate mentor, he was invited to join the new College of Chiropractors and was one of the first chiropractors ever to be included in the prestigious publication Dr. Fosters Guide. He went on to establish a birth trauma clinic at his private practice, caring for midwives, mums and babies, from King's College Hospital in South London. His research into the mind-body link gained him qualifications in sports psychology, NLP, hypnotherapy and a leap into the world of quantum physics, shamanism, and the wisdom of Huna.

A recipient of an honorary Doctor of Divinity, Kevin has been researching shamanism, metaphysics and the healing arts of the Pacific Islands. While in the US and Hawaii he has been fortunate to meet Pacific Island shamans, kahunas and massage masters. All have been willing to share their knowledge of lomilomi, Huna, and the aloha spirit. Kevin has participated in various shamanic practices, sweat lodges and vision quests. He has traveled the world, run marathons, competed in endurance events, holds a Black Belt in karate, and in the 1980s he set up the Streetwise self-defence course for women.

Kevin is an active fundraiser for charities supporting children's hospices and the founder of Azura, a voluntary O'hana who are dedicated to bringing smiles and laughter to seriously and terminally ill children, an interest activated by the infant death of his firstborn.

His wish is now to share a lifetime's collection of knowledge and techniques with the next generation: *"I am just a guy who likes to share what he knows."* With the support of the guardians, and after 40 years in development, Starlite® lomi was born, a beautiful lomi bodycare system, designed for lomilomi massage therapists. And in true aloha spirit, all Starlite® workshops, courses and individual treatments will raise awareness and funds for the Starlight® Children's Foundation.

> *"Kevin is an unassuming, likeable, down to earth guy, who believes that 'the message is far more important than the messenger' which is very refreshing in these days of self-publicity and celebrity."* - Kris

However ~ while in Hawaii he was given a piece of wisdom from an elder, who said that

> *"in order for Westerners to hear the message, they need to know about the authenticity of the messenger."*

So this is his story ~ let it be told!!

Foreword

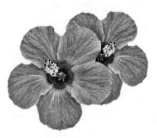

"Why me? I am nothing special, I am not famous, I am not an expert, and I am not even a native of the islands, so why me?"

I have known Kevin for many years and I know that this is a question he often struggled with for a long period of time.

I would say: "Why not him?"

Over time we both have learned to trust the guidance of the universe, he has pursued his own quest with great tenacity, a strength not seen in many. I know many westerners would have exploited the situation and betrayed the trust of the guardians; motivated by greed, they would have claimed the sacred knowledge as their own.

I also believe that a native of the islands would have been too near and too involved with the subject matter, influenced by history, ancestors and lineage. By choosing Kevin and not revealing the existence of lomilomi and Huna to him for 30 years, the keepers of the secrets ensured a total commitment and a non-biased development of their knowledge.

The fact that he has written this book and developed the Rainbow Course which teaches the Starlite® bodycare system demonstrates the right choice was made. However, his biggest achievement to date is Azura, a voluntary philanthropic O'hana, whose aim is to bring smiles and laughter to children with life-threatening or life-limiting illness by using the bodycare system to raise funds for the Starlight® Children's Foundation.

With a western scientifically based education he is able to present the spiritual, mystic and magical healing arts of the Pacific Islands to a new generation of westerners seeking answers beyond their material world. I believe that he is just one of a number of transformationals here on earth at this most historic of times. The fact that he sees himself as just another average guy is yet another reason that he was chosen for this project.

Kevin has been working in private practice for over 40 years; he has 'walked his talk' day after day, and year after year. Only now after a long career in physical therapy does he feel qualified enough to share his experience and knowledge.

Kevin has a unique way of sharing; he makes the complicated seem simple. He demystifies medical terminology and talks to you in everyday terms. He will often make fun of himself and empowers the student to explore the world of knowledge beyond his knowing.

If you are interested in complementary therapy, energy, spiritualism, shamanism, Huna, lomilomi or personal growth then I highly recommend this book to you. If you want a little taste of aloha, visit his website, book a course and meet the man that I am proud to call my friend.

Mrs L. Wright
- retired physiotherapist, London 2013

Preface

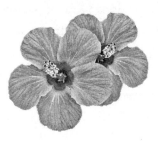

This book is about various elements of the universe coming together to create a new beginning at a precise moment in time. Stardate 21st December 2012 was the end of a 26,000-year cycle for human consciousness.

Unwittingly, for the last 40 years I have played my part in preparing for the new dawn that awaits humanity.

As a result of a life-changing knee injury in 1970, I was introduced to the world of the healing arts, complementary and conventional therapy. I have had a career in physical therapy that has taken me around the globe and given me the opportunity to meet many teachers – some famous, many not so famous, some embodied, some in spirit form. All have been mentors and have shared their wisdom with me; many of these can be found in the bibliography at the back of this book and to those who are interested in the subject matter, I would highly recommend further reading of the inspirational books that can be found in that listing.

What awaited me was a 40-year quest, a gathering of information, therapy techniques and wisdom. This would eventually blend together to reveal a bodycare system as ancient as the stars, but also as eternal as the universe.

This book is presented in two parts: in the first I wish to share some of my adventures and lessons with you, and introduce you to my helpers, guardians and friends on whose behalf I have been working. This part of the book is about personal growth leading to the discovery revealed in part two. In the second part of the book you can get a taste for the Starlite® bodycare system and experience its effect with a few guided exercises. At this stage I must emphasise that I am merely the messenger; the techniques, the wisdom and the message found within the Starlite® bodycare system are not mine, they belong to the spiritual ancestors of the oceanic people.

For my part, I am eternally grateful to have been shown the way of aloha. And it's in that spirit that I embrace my future role of sharing the beauty of the Starlite® bodycare system with those who love life, complementary therapy and the magic of aloha.

I hope you enjoy your read.

Mahalo and blessings.

Kevin

Dove Cottage, West Sussex 2013

Acknowledgements

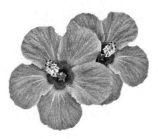

I would like to say a big thank you and Mahalo.

To the guardians of the beautiful Hawaiian Islands for introducing, blessing and sharing the aloha spirit with me and the world.

To all my teachers, trainers and students over the last half century, who are far too numerous to mention by name.

To Lisbet who introduced me to the world of physiotherapy and massage. To Leon Chaitow whose bodywork knowledge still amazes me. To everyone at the MCC and the FA Sports Medicine Centre. To Serge Kahili King for his insight into Huna. To Harry Uhane Jim and Tom Cochran for their beautiful adaptation of lomilomi. To Hank Wesselman who continues to expand my mind with his shamanic wisdom.

To Mindy and all at Panoma Press for their help and support in producing this book.

To my new family the Azura O'hana and their support of my vision.

To my parents Derek and Wendy who gave me the freedom to explore my own spiritual direction.

To Rob and Kay, close friends and family, who share my love of traveling. To my in-laws Fred and Brenda who have always treated me like a son.

To my children Darren and Natalie and their spouses Steph and Matt.

To my grandchildren Abigail and Isabelle, you make my world complete.

Finally, to the most precious person in my universe ~ Sandra. You are my wife, my best friend, my lover and my soul mate; in short, you are my life. Thank you for giving me three beautiful children, your support and your love, and for sharing this life's journey with me, I love you more than you can ever imagine.

Mahalo and blessings.
Kevin 2013

Part One

STARLiTE
The Secret Lomi

Discovering the sacred touch of aloha

Part One

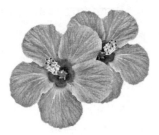

1:1 Introduction

On a dark summer's night many years ago, a young boy lay in the grass looking up at the stars dancing on a cosmic canvas; he stroked his dog and said: "If only I could..."

This book belongs to the elders and ancestors of Hawaii who have been guiding my steps for many years, before revealing their existence and my destiny. Every attempt has been taken to treat lomilomi, Huna and the oceanic people with the utmost respect. It is my sincere and humble hope that by bringing to light the wisdom of the elders, a drop of aloha will fall to earth and set in motion a new growth, perhaps one day that drop will turn to a shower and then to a cascade, a rainbow cascade of love, light and healing.

I have spent many years on self-development – physically, mentally and emotionally. However, a few years ago it struck me that no matter how much I improved myself, only one person benefited – but if I could influence other people in a positive way, that would make my life more meaningful. Over time, my interests shifted from developing talent for sports to a larger arena: developing talent for living. This I did by way of the healing arts. I have traveled the world and studied many systems of complementary therapy and human development. I have been 'walking this book' all my life and writing it for over ten years, therefore you may find that some paragraphs or pages will reflect the level of understanding I had at the precise moment that it was written, which may or may not reflect my current understanding.

Imagine driving along a road, a road you have never been on before. You don't know where this road leads to, or even the various places it will stop at on the way. What's more, you are traveling this road in the dark at night; your headlamps can only reveal the next few meters on your journey. You have no idea what the next place will reveal or even look like until you get there. Each day as you travel you gain knowledge and understanding and only when you reach the next destination does it then reveal its hidden beauty to you.

Such has my life journey been as I traveled on the road of the healing arts, starting with my feet firmly on planet earth, safe in the world of matter, western science and physical therapy. The road would pass through many lands and I would see many different landscapes; sometimes I would stop and take in the beauty of a place, learn its culture and discover its secrets. There have been times when this stopover has lasted for a few years, other times it's just a blink of an eye before I have moved on. But on each and every occasion I have found and collected 'golden nuggets' of knowledge, insight and information. Often this knowledge would be just a few grains of dust, magical stardust that collectively would eventually become a nugget of pure gold.

Once in a while I would find myself parked in a dark place, a place where I had to reach deep inside to find a light in order to take the next step forward. At times like these the learning can be profound, and gradually you learn to trust, trust in yourself, but more importantly trust in the universe, trust in the Divine.

I was to travel extensively through the physical realm, then deep into the world of metaphysics and spiritualism. The land of the shaman is truly mind-blowing, or more accurately mind-expanding, and its interblending with quantum physics was quite unexpected and an exciting surprise.

From where I stand now, I can see that this road is more than a road; it's more of a pathway, a magical pathway that bridges and connects the physical realm to that of the spiritual, a rainbow bridge.

This spiritual path leads to a portal, a stargate found right at the edge of eternity; here, if you can see through the veil of illusion, an infinite world of enchantment, love, light and magic awaits... on a road that never ends.

I am not a guru, I am not a kahuna, and I am not a teacher, for you are your own best teacher. I am just a guy who likes to share what he knows; I am here to speak my truth, it may not be your truth, but it is mine and in it I find my authenticity and authority to deliver the message.

In this book I will share with you some of my experiences 'in their raw form'; I'd like you to see what I saw and feel what I felt, then draw your own conclusions. I will introduce you to an ancient healing art form that is destined for a new dawn; I will also share with you my heartfelt wish for the future.

So come, walk with me as a friend and fellow traveler, take each baby step together and let me show you the sights. Where are we going?

The answer to that question, my friend, is up to you.

As one prominent quantum scientist once said: "It all depends on how far down the rabbit hole you want to go..."

Pieces of puzzles make up a key, unlocking a clue to set you free.

No path is straight for they all take a bend, to spiral around starting over again.

All things above are like that below; the greater it is the smaller you go.

So quiet your head and follow your heart; the spiral – a circle – comes back to the start.

A doorway opens that's always been sealed, secrets and mysteries finally revealed...

1:2 The Puzzle

Once upon a time when the world was full of magic, awe and wonder, there was a land, a land of light, peace and beauty, a land that was home to the descendants of star travelers. These people had learned the secrets of embodiment and the preservation of the physical human form, their earth vehicle. This great knowledge and wisdom was woven into the tapestry of consciousness and used for the benefit of all.

Then one day and with no warning there was a wobble of the earth, the great land was destroyed in a single night, torn asunder by earthquakes, smashed to pieces by titanic tidal waves, blown apart by volcanic eruptions. Very few of the original 'starmen' survived the cataclysm which pulverized their ancient civilization.

The consciousness of knowledge was blown apart into 50,000 pieces, like a giant jigsaw. It was swept up by whirlwinds into the stratosphere, many fragments traveled a cosmic wave into infinity, others circled the globe gliding on various trade winds. Eventually, after many years, the winds eased and the jigsaw of knowledge settled on land and sea, drifting on currents to the ends of the earth.

Every now and then over the next 10,000 years or so, an unsuspecting traveler would come across a piece of the puzzle, a single seed of wisdom, and a new body of knowledge would be born. Cultures in lands as far apart as China, India, Egypt and Mexico have all used similar healing methods. Descendants of the few survivors traveled the vast oceans; for thousands of years they took the remnants of their great knowledge with them. These descendants left seeds across the ocean; eventually, after many attempts to establish a home on islands across the Pacific, they settled on the Marquesas and then the Hawaiian Islands. While thousands of pieces of the puzzle lay hidden under the earth or within the layers of sediment on the sea bed, some remained hidden, often in plain sight.

Over the last 100 years or so, high guardians have been brought into this world, soul seeds, individuals who are ready to experience the magic of this ancient knowledge. Pieces of the puzzle are working their way to the surface and being found on a regular basis.

"These 'transformationals' come from every community, and at every social level. It is they who may set in motion a golden age for humanity for the next 2,000 years." - Hank Wesselman

Many moons ago, a young boy was given a piece of the great puzzle, passed down by another torch bearer just before she disembodied and returned to spirit. The unsuspecting youngster held in his hand a key to an adventure that would take him around the world and into the infinite dimensions of the dreamtime. He would fly the skies of the earth and surf the waves of the cosmos. His quest was to find the adjoining pieces and complete one small part of a great picture; this quest would take over 40 years.

The young boy pursued his quest with the enthusiasm and energy of a young tiger pursuing his prey. Each day the beast required feeding, he would be constantly on the lookout for pieces of the puzzle and once in a while he would stumble upon a golden nugget. There would be many false leads and disappointments, but just when all seemed lost, and often in the most unexpected places, the glitter of treasure caught his eye and yet another piece would be added.

With great tenacity and perseverance, the young boy cub, who was now a young man, would seek knowledge and healing techniques from the people of the earth. His quest would take him to large cities and remote islands, from the deserts of middle earth to the land of ice and fire.

As his collection of puzzle pieces became bigger and bigger a picture started to emerge, a picture of massage, bodywork and healing techniques, coupled with the knowledge of how to use them and the wisdom of when to use them. Then one day he decided to share his small section of the puzzle, but many felt threatened and were not interested. "Why become a beginner when I can stay as an expert?" they said. They wanted to stay safe in their comfort zones and massage their own egos.

The young man, who was now a man of many summers, understood that the world was not yet ready and the secret of the puzzle would not yet be revealed. Maybe, just maybe, this would take more than just one lifetime, he thought, as he returned to the path of adventure and discovery.

As more and more pieces began to emerge, the finding of them became harder. Trying to find the authentic ancient nugget amongst the now many copies was akin to looking for one special tree in a vast forest. Over the years, others had also found pieces of the puzzle, but not all understood the value of their find. Some would see a business opportunity, produce cheap copies and market it as their own. In turn, others would copy the copies and yet another tree was planted, hiding the authentic original in plain sight, but out of view to the thousands of eyes that could not see.

Unperturbed, the man of many summers ventured into the dark woods, looking, always looking. But now he had developed a sense of hearing, and with intuition and concentration, he could hear the faint whisper of an ancient secret wanting to be heard.

Then one cold winter's night during the darkest of times, when life itself seemed to be waning, he was sitting alone, lost in the dark forest, cold, tired and carrying yet another sack full of potential techniques that needed sifting through just in case it held a small handful of stardust. For, you see, some of the original pieces had now been fractured, broken up and mixed with a man-made concoction, in order to feed the drug habit of the new age. Unable to find the pathway back to the light, and for the first time since starting his quest, on this moonless night the man of many summers and one dark winter asked the question: Why?

"Trust me," said the soft voice, "follow the star." On that dark winter's night he had fallen asleep, but was he asleep or was he awake, was he in the physical world or that of the dreamtime? "Trust me," the voice said again, "follow the star," whispered the voice. He adjusted his vision to the dark shadows of the forest and there in the distance was a twinkle a small glitter in the twilight. With reinvigorated energy he set off in the direction indicated. Many days and nights passed before he eventually arrived at a dead-end; disappointed, he sat down at the water's edge. Believing that he had made a mistake in choosing that direction, he decided to retrace his steps and then move forward again. He had only traveled for a few days but the return journey was long and arduous – it took many months before he arrived back.

Then one day in the corner of his eye there was a twinkle, the direction and route forward looked the same but somehow it was different. Once again he stepped into the unknown. Follow the star, he thought as he headed deep into the woods. After several days of hard toil he arrived at yet another dead-end. He slumped on to a boulder, disappointed but not surprised.

He reasoned that it must be an optical illusion, a mirage, a trick of the mind, there was no star to follow, and if only he could get back to his western scientific way of thinking, then the way forward would become obvious. Two more years passed and the man of many summers and three dark winters was still lost in the woods, the path was slow and tough, he was sinking in mud due to the weight that he was carrying. It had been another long hard day and he had traveled but a few feet; tired, despondent and ready to give up, he curled up for the night. "I wish," he said as he closed his eyes, "I wish I could have another chance to follow the star." In his bones and to the very core of his being he knew that it was the right thing to do.

"Trust me," said the familiar voice, "you must leave everything behind and follow the star." In that moment he made a determined commitment to do whatever was required, without question or complaint and without his overriding western cultural need to know the outcome beforehand. With that commitment he found himself floating in a liquid of blue energy, at least it felt like a liquid, much like a lava lamp. There were sparks of light, and bubbles dancing in the blue fluid. A bubble of light developed into a soft wispy female face, a face so full of love and compassion that the man of many summers and three dark winters began to cry. Tears of happiness were followed by a smile of knowing, a knowing that he was looking into the very heart of creation through the eyes of Azura, the star of twilight.

This jigsaw was unlike any other, the pieces were not cardboard cut-outs with a printed design on one side. The puzzle pieces were pieces of knowledge, pieces of wisdom, pieces of consciousness coming together to form a vibrating living energetic body. In the years that followed, its secrets would gently unfold like a flower in the sunlight to reveal a magic, a beauty beyond all expectations.

Then out of the blue a lightning bolt hit him right between the eyes, a true satori moment and as time itself stood still, he received visits, friends of Azura, spirits of the ocean. His new purpose became clear, he was to take his collection of ancient wisdom, futuristic healing techniques that were once stardust at the time of creation, and share them with the new 'children of the rainbow'. These spirits who travel the earth with aloha in their hearts would find him – 'when the teacher is ready the students will arrive'.

The man of many summers and three dark winters was no more; he had been rejuvenated and once again he was able to bounce about like a young tiger but with the advantage of wisdom, of age, and experience. Although still embodied, he appeared to the dream world as an old gray wolf, someone who was ready to share what he had learned, he was ready to teach those who would listen.

The next day, feeling as light as a feather, he set off in the direction he had seen the night before and, in less than a second, was out of the dark forest and on to a beautiful island beach where he enjoyed the welcoming display of a young female dolphin playing in the surf. When she had finished playing, she gently rolled on to her side and looked toward the shore... those eyes! Could it be...?

> *"Think like a man of action,*
> *Act like a man of thought."*
>
> Henri Bergson

1:3 Life-changing injury

The blue lights had just disappeared down the lane. Mark and his broken leg had been safely transferred from the football pitch into the ambulance and the 16 year-old physio had been congratulated for the professional way he handled the situation. I looked at the scene and asked: "How did I get to here?"

It all started six months earlier when my life was turned upside down and everything changed. The date was Easter 1970 and my future had been planned out; like every schoolboy, the dream was to play professional football. I had already trialed at a top London club and knew that I would not make the grade; however, I was determined to play at a decent level; at this young age, football was my life.

I loved sports; my day would always start early delivering the morning newspapers, we had been taught to support ourselves from an early age with any little money that we could earn. It was then a quick trip home for breakfast, I would cycle the five miles to school and go into early morning circuit training before the first lesson of the day. Most days would contain some sort of sporting activity and I could always be found on the playing fields during break/recess. After school it was back to the gym or a cross-country run; I had recently been selected to represent Croydon schools at the national cross-country competition.

Since the age of five, after being taken to the Royal Military Tournament held at Earls Court, London, I had ambitions of joining the Royal Marines and becoming a physical training instructor. There was now less than six months to go before this was to happen.

Then 'bang!' I was kicked in the knee whilst playing around with a football in a local park – not even in a competitive match. It was early evening and light was fading fast, I picked up my bike and limped home, two miles uphill. By the time I got home my knee was throbbing; I sat on the sofa and rested my leg. In those days we didn't even know about the advantages of ice. This was followed by a restless night, I just could not get comfortable and my knee was burning hot. When I woke up the next morning it was with a knee that was red, inflamed, painful, and the size of a football – it was as if someone had pumped it up with air during the night.

There was to be the normal three-hour-long wait at the hospital A&E as the doctors attended the last of the Saturday night/Sunday morning party revelers. Then it was my turn. I was sent to the x-ray department and then taken back to a cubicle where I was introduced to an Indian doctor; he appeared complete with turban, beard and a big smile. He explained that I had torn part of the patella tendon (part of the thigh muscle that houses the kneecap and stabilizes the knee) and I had also ruptured the cruciate ligament (found deep in the knee joint) which in turn had filled the capsule around the knee joint with blood and synovial fluid. He said that the first thing to do was to address the pain by reducing the swelling; he then pulled out the biggest syringe that I had ever seen. I immediately thought it was an elephant syringe and the doctor had a good sense of humor. It took a few minutes before I realised, this was no joke...

Have you ever seen a horror film where a person is wired up to a machine and his energy is being painfully extracted, bit by bit, from his body? Well, that's exactly what it felt like. This large needle was pushed into my swollen knee and the syringe was sucking my energy, my very life essence was being drained from me, or at least that's how it felt. In reality it was the mixture of blood and synovial fluid that was being removed from my swollen joint.

I was so pleased it was over that I didn't care about the fact that I would be in plaster for six weeks and then there were to be several months of rehab; the realization that my pending career and future dreams had been shattered had not yet hit me. You see, in London in 1970 there was no keyhole surgery that would allow a patient to be in and out of hospital the same day. The choice was to have full open surgery to repair the rupture, exposing the joint to possible infection, or to manage the injury by a conservative approach. Either way, I would never play football at the same level again or reach the required level of physical fitness to be an instructor in the Forces. The doctors chose the latter option and my leg was plastered.

After six weeks the plaster was removed and I was a 16-year-old with the leg the size of a nine year-old's. Not only did it look like a stick that had been attached to my body, but I could not bend the knee one degree; rehab was going to be a long, long slog.

Rehabilitation

My local hospital in South London was in the process of revamping and upgrading its physiotherapy department (physical therapy); as a result, a number of the physios had been reassigned to other hospitals during the works. The few that were left concentrated on cardiac recovery and hip replacement, the latter being the big thing back then. The equipment available was for that purpose and, on top of that, their clinics were full. My injury was sports related and required a different rehab regime. To overcome this problem I was introduced to Lisbet, a retired physiotherapist of Swedish descent. She was in her seventies and was engaged on a part-time basis to help during this unusual period. Lisbet was a lot of fun, she had a lot of knowledge and an exquisite touch – apparently this had become more sensitive after she lost her sight. Now you would think that a 16-year-old boy and a 70-plus lady would have nothing in common, but we got on like a house on fire. She was about to introduce me to the world of anatomy, rehabilitation and to what was then considered a 'new age' treatment: Swedish massage.

Lisbet had an upright stance that the years had not diminished; she had shoulder-length gray hair and even though time had taken her sight there was still a twinkle in her eye. In her day she must have been quite a stunner. It was not long before I was calling her Ingrid – after the Hollywood actress Ingrid Bergman – and joked that she should have been an actress, not a physiotherapist. This would always put a smile on her face. I think she quite liked my light-hearted approach to life; I had a feeling that hers had been a much harder and more rigid way of life. She had a quirky personality: it was a bit of a mixture between a matron, which reflected her status and the pre-war period that she grew up in, and a relaxed new age approach to life. I expect she was the world's first hippy, possibly due to her upbringing in Sweden. She lived on her own in a small terraced house no more than half a mile from the hospital, and when I became a bit more mobile I would hobble round for a cup of tea and a chat about me, my goals and my family. She didn't reveal too much about herself, it was as though she had come to terms with her end of days and just wanted to hear about fresh young lives. Lisbet passed away about eight months after my rehab was completed; however she had passed on a lot of knowledge and had ignited a spark in me. Looking back, I suppose she saw me as her legacy. She had a great life story and I wanted to hear it. Now I, in turn, have reached a point in my life where I feel compelled to share my experience with those who have ears to hear.

Because I had been involved in sport and fitness all my life, I had a pretty good understanding of how my body worked, or so I thought. My rehab program was comprehensive and because I was interested in the process and was always questioning how things were done and why they worked, Lisbet would explain everything in minute detail. I was living and learning about injury rehab every minute of every day – it was a real intimate experience. Lisbet even asked a colleague to show me the new isometric exercise machines that were being installed in the new physio department and he took his time to explain about each machine in detail. You must remember that this was 1970; there were no gyms, spas or personal trainers, aerobics and fitness classes were still years away. I was just a schoolboy and had access to what was then state-of-the-art equipment; I was even asked to demonstrate this equipment to Princess Anne when she arrived to open the new center.

During this period I took my first First Aid course with the British Red Cross and have regularly attended refresher workshops ever since. This is something that I would recommend to everyone everywhere, especially young parents. Within six months of passing this course I had successfully used the CPR (Cardiopulmonary Resuscitation) and Heimlich maneuver techniques to save lives. I spent one very enjoyable year as a life guard where First Aid knowledge is required on a daily basis. The same skills have helped me look after football clubs, Scouts, my own children and members of the general public. The rewards are great when you have been able to help someone in need, when you have the confidence and self-assurance to take charge in terms of First Aid, after a road traffic accident or any other disaster. If you only attend one course in your life, let it be a First Aid course.

As my interest grew and my fitness returned, Lisbet introduced me to Swedish massage. As I stated earlier, this was seen as new age, and had only started to gain popular appeal (in the UK) after being used by hippies in the 1960s; at this time sports massage was still something for the future. The spark had now turned into a fire, Lisbet could not have given me a better gift, it was a gift of love, and started a love affair with massage and bodywork that has lasted for nearly half a century.

Eight months after my injury, I returned to the football club – not as a player (I have played a few games since, but never at the same skill level) but armed with my new skills of First Aid, injury and rehab knowledge and the secret weapon of Swedish massage. I returned as the club's new physiotherapist.

Thank you Ingrid; if we had not shared that special period in time, my life would have been different and this book would have not been written. (Battersea Park, London, 1980)

A picture began to unfold
That revealed a secret once told
Techniques and knowledge was advanced
Practitioners and followers of the Stardance

1:4 The Quest

In the story of King Arthur and the Knights of the Round Table, the quest of the knights was to search for and find the Holy Grail, the chalice that was used at the Last Supper. The knights would leave Camelot and go on lifelong adventures seeking this elusive treasure; those adventures still continue and the chalice still remains out of reach. However, the real treasure was to be found in their adventure, the journey itself revealed many golden nuggets, each unveiling its own treasure as a step towards enlightenment for the knight who discovered it.

Unknowingly, following my introduction to massage and bodywork in 1970 I also had embarked on a lifelong quest seeking golden nuggets, special techniques, secret knowledge and the way of the light.

Although I had been practicing my physical art for a few years, my true pathway became a lot clearer to me after completing a sports massage course at St. Mary's Sports College in Twickenham, the home of English rugby. Our tutor was also the massage therapist for the national team and we students would often be working on the players after their training sessions. As part of the final assessment we had to assess and massage members of the public in open clinic. Unlike the players, the public did not turn up just needing a massage; often their presenting condition required muscle stretching, joint mobilisation, and other soft tissue work that left the students frustrated because they did not have the skills to give a comprehensive treatment. It was from their frustrations that I knew I needed to develop a holistic, non-diagnostic bodywork system specially designed for massage therapists.

By this time I had gained over ten years' experience of collecting bodywork techniques from any course or workshop that appeared. As various sports injury and massage associations came into existence, I would be first in – soaking up all the information and techniques on offer, much like a sponge soaks up all the available water. It was during this period that I started to formulate a new and comprehensive bodywork system. At this point I must make it clear that this was not a system developed by me, I was merely collecting all the golden nuggets being exposed by the universe and following guidance from the same source. I started to choreograph a new dance, and new ways of using old techniques that the universe had given to me and others in time gone by.

So my quest was now clear, or was it?

Looking back with the advantage of future knowledge, I can now see and understand the path that the universe had lit up, step by step, and the direction I had been guided in, but this was often a confusing pathway. I was being driven to attend workshops and was collecting techniques at a phenomenal rate. On many occasions I would attend a weekend workshop only to find that the technique being taught varied only slightly from one I already knew. Often this turned out to be because the 'founder' either could not do the original technique or simply wanted to change it enough to call it their own. On one particular occasion, the teacher had changed the technique she was taught from a right-handed technique to a left-handed technique, simply because she was left-handed, and thus 'discovered' a new therapy. Over the years, I've found that complementary therapy tends to attract good people with kind hearts, but on the flip-side, and at a higher level, it can also be rife with politics and egos.

For many years I had this overwhelming sense of direction, collecting techniques in order to form soft tissue bodywork for massage therapy, but only a vague view of what to do with the detail. The analogy is like putting together a 10,000 piece jigsaw puzzle without knowing what the picture looks like. Furthermore, all the pieces required to make this picture are mixed up in a container along with 10,000 more pieces all of the same size, shape, and similar photo detail. There were often times I would find and attach a piece only to discover later that it was the wrong piece and needed changing. The pieces of the jigsaw represent techniques and there was no rhyme, rhythm or sequence to when and how they would arrive. When I truly discovered one, I was ecstatic – it really was like finding a 'golden nugget' to add to the treasure trove that I was collecting.

The overpowering learning I received from this process was learning the art of patience and to trust and totally surrender to the universe, knowing that everything would be OK in its own time, and no pressure or wishing from me was going to hurry that up.

Workshops

I have been fortunate enough to have attended hundreds of workshops, lectures and courses in over 50 countries around the world. I have loved the travel, the joyous people I've met, and the variety of knowledge that has been passed on to me, and I can honestly say that I have learned something from every teacher I have ever met and from many of the other course participants. To every one of them I send a big Mahalo and blessings.

For me, the secret of attracting golden nuggets and extracting sacred information from courses is to approach each one as though it's your first. As a Zen master would say, you should be like an empty cup. It's simple, but not easy.

Think back to your very first workshop, course, or therapy – you were open to every thought, every suggestion, and receptive to every technique taught. You would soak up the information offered, often without question. This then became a foundation on which you could build, it became a core belief and set a standard by which you would judge other workshops, courses and teachers. Unfortunately, often human nature and ego start to get in the way.

Do we approach the next new therapy or workshop with the same beginner's mind? No way.

We are so desperate not to be seen as a beginner or a rookie that we use our limited knowledge gained from the first workshop to criticize, judge or undermine what's being taught; we often then compare the two different therapies. How many of us during our personal introduction at the start of a workshop rattle on about how much we know, how good we are, how many qualifications we have? At this time, right at the beginning of the workshop, the ego sets the scene. Have you ever considered the repercussions of this approach?

A teacher faced with someone with real or perceived greater knowledge or more experience may feel threatened and uncomfortable. This may result in a lack of confidence, or in a slight aggression as they try to gain control in their position as head of the workshop, which they might see as being under threat. They may challenge you as a person, or your depth of knowledge, by trying to make you look small, which is another way of regaining their perceived loss of power. There are teachers who will accept you as a peer. Either way, the result is the same: their teaching approach to you and your learning approach to the workshop will change, for once you are in this position you cannot operate with a beginner's mind and the teacher will not teach you as a beginner. Of course we are not talking about world-class teachers, masters of their trade who have evolved past this level; unfortunately this equates to a very small number of enlightened individuals.

I have experienced this situation, both personally and by watching others; at the time I understood the problem but not how to deal with it. This was one of my first lessons in trusting the universe; one night I simply asked the universe for guidance and then went to sleep. In the early days I had developed an ego; I was a teenager with some very special skills that are recognised and appreciated by others. This was a potent mix for an inflated ego and, looking back, some of my first workshops were embarrassing with the ego running loose. I would get frustrated and upset if the workshop then failed to give me what I needed. But I now understand that this period was also a very important learning experience for me and I will never forget the lessons from the universe. I was asked: "What do you want from the workshops?" And the answer came: "I wanted the teacher to give me the pure essence of the therapy he or she was teaching." And from that I could extract the golden nuggets. I then asked how I get the teacher to give me this. The answer was instant: "Become a beginner, approach each experience with a beginner's mind."

I would no longer approach a workshop from the point of view of ego. From that day on I became like a chameleon blending into the background, becoming just another student doing nothing that would stand out. When asked about my experience, I was economical with the truth and just said that I had some massage experience. I was not a beginner and it would be untruthful to claim to be, also many workshops required a level of experience. I found that by approaching each workshop at the minimum experience level I could give myself the freedom to learn and the teacher the freedom to teach with no pressure on either of us. I was not a beginner but over the years I developed a beginner's mind.

I am simply a human being with all the normal inadequacies, including that of ego. However, with the support of my chameleon helper I am able to suppress the ego during workshops. Fortunately for me, I have always been a good listener; I love to hear about the life stories of others, but I am not so good when talking about my experiences, so writing this book is a trip beyond my comfort zone. In opening myself up, I make myself vulnerable, defenceless, the complete opposite of the protective shell I've had all my adult life. So why do it? Simply, it needs to be done

We are now in transition between what was and what will be, and the decisions that we make or don't make today will affect the entire next stage of human evolution, a truly awesome responsibility.

Hank Wesselman

1:5 The Gatekeeper

When I was a teenager I would often be out jogging and one route would take me down a country lane – it was more like an unmade track used by a few horse riders and walkers. At one point it dissected a piece of woodland: to the left was a hedgerow just over waist height and in the middle of the hedgerow, about one meter back from the track, was an old broken wooden gate. It was a bar-type gate and the overgrown long grass on the other side poked through and over the gate; the gate appeared to be an entrance to what was a long forgotten track leading into a dark and mysterious part of the woods. Sitting on a log in the shadows just in front of the gate was an old man; he was always sitting there, hunched back and with a hood pulled over his head. He seemed to just stare at the ground and he took no notice of any travelers running, walking or riding past and they in turn did not seem to notice him.

One day when I was passing this spot again I happened to notice that the old man wasn't there; I had gotten so used to seeing him that it felt out of kilter that he wasn't at home. I had never even spoken to the old man, but curiosity got the better of me and I stopped running, and then looked around for him. There was no sign of him and obviously no one had been the other side of the gate for many years. I then stood on the bottom wooden rail of the gate in order to gain a little height and tried to look into the wooded area. This, however, was hindered by the long grass, and so leaning slightly forward I gently parted the long grass with both hands and tried to focus on the dark overgrown vegetation behind.

As I looked I could see laid out before me a beautiful scene of a clearing in the woods with lush green grass, flowers, butterflies, bees and birds; there were lambs playing and a doe standing watching from the edge of the copse. The sunlight was streaking through the treetops reflecting a burst of rainbow light from raindrops on the leaves. Not quite believing what I saw, I closed my eyes tight and then opened them again; it was gone – the vision, the mirage whatever it was, it was gone.

I nearly fell from the gate in fright, there was someone behind me. Quickly turning around, I came face to face with the old man, or should I say face to hood with a black shadow beneath it, the sense and presence surrounding this cloaked figure was that of an old man, a very old man. "Who are you?" I said, and immediately the response came back, "I am the gatekeeper." The response was not through voice but through thought. "The gatekeeper, what do you do?" I said inquisitively.

"I wait," came the reply.

"For what?"

"For someone to open the gate." I was taken aback and remembered that I had seen this man sitting here every time that I ran past since using this track, and that had been almost three years.

"What do you want it open for? How long have you been waiting?"

"So many questions, I've been waiting a long time, a very long time and I would like it open so that I don't have to wait any more," came the reply.

By now I was convinced that the old man had lost his marbles, but I was happy to play along. "Well, I can open the gate, but first I'll have to cut back all of the overgrowth and clear the weeds before it will open."

"That's right," was not the response I expected, but as promised I returned the next day. Although the old man was not there, I cleared an area behind the gate and found what looked like a stepping stone. You know, I never did see the old man again, but I did return to explore the mystery beyond the gate.

Unbeknown to me at the time, that day and that stepping stone was the start of a 40-year quest to uncover the hidden pathway, step by step. It would lead me on an adventure far beyond the woods and deep into a magical valley where ancient mysteries and secrets lived. I would meet spirits and animals from other dimensions, have my beliefs, my perceptions and my truths turned upside down, wrung inside out, then be hung out to dry. I would be given an insight to a world that existed 18 million years ago, learn to ride cosmic waves using a 35,000-year-old philosophy that quantum science has only recently discovered, I would be taught the healing skills of the stardancers and find my purpose, my life's path for this incarnation.

There would be many setbacks, many hardships, many wrong turns and many adventures, but there has been much joy, much laughter, much happiness and a great deal of love along the way.

Only after I had completed 40 years of searching for each one of the golden nuggets of knowledge that would become the next piece of this 5D jigsaw of magic, only after clearing the overgrowth of the valley, cutting back the vegetation, unblocking the streams, cleaning the ponds, only after new life had returned to the valley, only when I had passed all the tests set before me, only then did she show me the hidden secrets found in the esoteric records of universal memory, the cosmic treasure, the ancient knowledge and wisdom and ultimately the true magic of the valley.

The time has come to listen to the echoes from our land; the ancient wisdom spoken in simple words and soft voices...

We have not heard them, because we have not taken the time to listen.

Perhaps now is the time to open our ears and our hearts...

1:6 Shamanism

I was formally introduced to shamanism while in Australia in the now normal unpredictable way. This was our second tour of Australia and on this trip we had been introduced to the aboriginal ways, first in Darwin in the Northern Territories followed by Didgeridoo's lesson at an aboriginal festival in Cairns in the tropical north of Queensland, and finally in the heart of aboriginal culture at Uluru (Ayers Rock) in the center of the country.

Now, though, we were enjoying a little 'downtime' on a beach in Western Australia. The sand was soft, the water cool and clear and the sun was very hot. It was one of those great lazy days of summer. When it was time for lunch we decided to visit a waterfront restaurant some 500 meters away that was surrounded by small shops. When my wife pointed this out, I couldn't help but notice the sun reflecting in a ray of white light from the glass of one of the shops. As we approached the shops it become apparent that it was a book shop and the reflection came not from the front window as I had assumed, but from inside. "Maybe a mirror," I said to no one in particular, and promptly gave it no more thought as my attention turned to the beautiful looking food in the beach-themed restaurant.

An hour or so later, after a great meal and a cold beer, we headed back to the beach passing the same shops as before. I was surprised to notice the sun still reflecting from something inside the book shop; my curiosity got the better of me and I popped inside for no other reason than to see the source of the reflection. To my surprise it was coming from a book cover. In this shop the books were stacked end-on in little pigeon holes; in front of them a single book had been turned face-on so that the shopper could see the front cover. This particular book had a silver foil face and was the source of the sun's reflection. *Way of Shamanism* by Leo Rutherford had me engrossed for the remainder of the trip. I had no idea what shamanism was about but purchased the book after only reading two lines: 'Shamanism is the oldest spiritual path on this planet, it is not a belief system it is a path of knowledge.'

To top it all, that afternoon while sitting on the beach reading the first chapters, a baby dolphin appeared just 25 meters offshore and swam around a small group of children playing in the water. If you believe in signs from the universe, then this surely was a good one.

As stated, this book was my 'formal' introduction to shamanism. I use the word formal because the more I read, and the more I studied, the more I realized that this was a subject that I knew a lot about. I have been having shamanic experiences all through my life. I just didn't know that they were called shamanic, I didn't even realize that others did not have the same experiences as I did. I simply thought what was normal for me applied to everyone else; after all, I reasoned, I was just ordinary therefore my natural instincts must also be ordinary. This realization brought with it mixed feelings: on one hand I was overjoyed to discover a treasure of talent, hidden to plain sight; on the other hand I was upset and a little frustrated to have missed opportunities, especially as a child, not to have used these gifts in a much more productive way.

Morphing

We all have these talents, but some are more developed than others, so why did I not recognize them as enhanced or special talents? Let me explain with this childhood example of everyday use of shamanic talents. After school my friends and I would head off to the park for a game of football/soccer, we would split into two teams and name our team after a professional club. We would then name ourselves after our favorite player. If I was a striker I may have chosen Jimmy Greaves, a small genius who could dribble with the ball, beating player after player and then he stroked the ball into the net; or Bobby Charlton who had a cannonball kick; or if I was playing midfield I would choose someone like Alan Mulley who was solid as a rock. Now each player had different personalities and distinctive body movements; I would now morph myself into my chosen player based on my limited knowledge of that player. Back in the 1960s we had very little TV access and would only see glimpses of matches; we did, however, go to many live games and this helped to get a 'feeling' for the player. Often in the game that followed I felt as though I was in the player's body, behaving the way he would, and moving the way he would. If I was Jimmy Greaves, I would often go on a similar run, dribbling the ball and stroking the ball into the net; I would feel my body moving as his appeared to move, this I knew because it was different from my own natural movements. On the occasion that I was Bobby Charlton I could kick the ball with more power than I had before – this would totally surprise my friends who didn't see me as having a strong shot. Until I read the book on shamanism I assumed that the other boys were doing exactly the same when they 'became' a famous player. However, I now know from recent enquiries that my morphing experience was not replicated by the other players.

This is very similar to the actions of impersonators, who mimic facial expressions, body movements and the voices of famous people; often we even mistake them for the real thing.

If there are kids out there with this ability, you have a special talent – try and develop it. I, for instance, never took this skill into a competitive match; it was merely something we did to have fun after school. Now this could be a fun experiment to do, one that I believe could work. Try to morph into a player on a daily basis, keep practicing hour after hour and eventually you should build muscle memory which will then allow you to take on board the player's skills as your own. Keep repeating this process with each skill set that you require and you can become a composite player made up of a number of skills from more than one person. After all 'there are no limits'.

"True magic is the act in which the ones practicing it can step into the spirit worlds, the worlds of things hidden, where they may enhance their personal mana with unlimited power that resides there, and then they may use their enhanced mana to manifest into this world here through conscious awareness. This is the way all magic happens." - Hale Makua

The best and most beautiful things

Must be felt with the heart...

1:7 Introduction to Lomilomi

By the new millennium I had collected nearly all the pieces of the bodywork jigsaw and was in the process of building the picture of the jigsaw. I had no idea of what the picture would look like when it was finished. I knew that there were two things missing: one was the right massage for pre- and post-bodywork treatment and the second was something elusive, a philosophy maybe, a something that I simply referred to as 'the magic', for without 'the magic' I only had a collection of techniques. By now I had learned to trust the universe, go with the flow, safe in the knowledge that something would show up when the time was right.

As mentioned in a previous chapter, I was introduced to the world of shamanism in Australia some years before. Since then my study and practice of shamanism had opened up a whole new dimension for me. But still I had to keep it a secret from my chiropractic colleagues and patients. Shamanic principles felt natural to me and I had realized early on that I had been using shamanism all my life, it was just simply not identified as that.

I felt like a coin: the 'head' side was my public face, it was what I was recognized by, it was the same 'face' as the rest of society. And when that side of the coin was facing up, no one could see my private and more interesting 'tail' side. And so it was, until my wife decided to book a vacation to the Hawaiian Islands. Now I love traveling, and when I go to another country I always pick up an 'eye witness' travel book as background study of the people, the history and interesting locations. This time I had two books and they had been packed for me; to my surprise, one book was titled Huna – Hawaiian shamanism. The computer had picked up on two points of interest – Hawaii and shamanism – and this had resulted in the purchase of the book I was now holding. I just hoped that there would be time to read it as our vacation was jam-packed with things to do and places to go.

We spent the next ten days island-hopping and the Huna book remained closed.

Then on the last day of our vacation I was relaxing in the hotel bar after dinner; everyone in our group had gone to their rooms to finish packing before our trip home first thing in the morning. This was the first time that I had an opportunity to open the book on Huna. The next three hours passed in the blink of an eye, and then something magical happened, the next chapter read: Lomilomi Hawaiian Shamanic Massage – whaaaaaaaaaat!!

Was this the missing link? Was this the rim of my coin that would join both sides, both aspects of me, together? Well, there was no stopping me, it was now 1am and I was at the hotel reception booking a lomilomi massage for first thing in the morning and at 7am I was on the massage table experiencing lomilomi for the first time in my life.

It was a long journey home – five hours to the US mainland and a further 11 hours to London. We were tired and I was deflated; what had promised to be the magical missing link had turned out to be just another very ordinary massage, and by the time I arrived home I was not sure if it was the quality of the massage or whether my expectations were just too high. Still, looking on the bright side I had found Huna; this without a doubt was the missing philosophy I was looking for, and would give me plenty to explore and study in the years ahead.

In the weeks that followed my return to the UK, I researched lomilomi, found books, articles and websites; everything I read was opposite to my experience. I started to make enquiries and contacted a number of teachers around the world. I had decided that it was wrong to judge a therapy on one disappointing experience; I, more than anyone, should know that you can teach a technique to several people and every one of them will have a different touch. Therefore I reasoned the only way of truly experiencing and understanding lomilomi was to treat it like any other therapy and attend a workshop. Now I was in luck, there was one being held in Brighton the following weekend and it was only 50 miles away. I booked my place on the workshop and on a cold dark December morning I was driving into my future. With all my desire I wanted this massage called lomilomi to be my missing link – after all, I had all the techniques and the philosophy, what was missing was a special massage therapy.

In over 40 years of complementary health study I have attended hundreds of workshops, in every corner of the world. These days, when I attend a workshop I keep my expectations low and would call a workshop successful if I find just one or – heavens above! – two 'golden nuggets' of information or techniques that I can add to my ever-growing jigsaw of bodywork therapy. I can honestly say that I have learned something from every teacher, and after three days in Brighton I had learned that if I wanted to study lomilomi I had to return to the States. And for that insight I am eternally grateful.

Six months later I was on a plane flying to Florida, returning to a therapy that had let me down twice and was something I had never done before – was I mad? Now, at this point I must say that something was just not right. Everything that I had read and continued to read about lomilomi made me believe that I was on the right track. I had narrowed my research down and targeted one person in particular who had inspired me with a sacred version of lomilomi. I was enjoying a cold beer at 10,000 feet thinking I bet he doesn't know that as far as I am concerned, lomilomi is now on trial, and I was expecting failure – after all, a leopard does not change its spots.

Over the years I have developed a workshop persona, I call him 'the chameleon'. The objective is to retrieve information, techniques and golden nuggets wherever and whenever I can find them. And I have found that the best way to achieve this is to be egoless and non-threatening (discard all professional titles, qualifications and experience) and to be open to a new or different way (approach each workshop as a beginner). This allows you to be yourself, without ego, without having to prove anything, without having to live up to expectations. It allows room for mistakes as you learn using a beginner's mind, or in the world of Zen Buddhism 'come forth like an empty cup'. It also allows the teacher to be themselves, without feeling under pressure to perform, or feel judged; the best way to teach, I believe, is also without ego.

To all of my teachers, and there have been hundreds – some famous, many not so famous, some still embodied and many returned to spirit – to all of my teachers, I thank you, and at the same time ask you to forgive my non-disclosure. My only intention was to experience the purity of your expression. In my defence I say that I am a collector of techniques and information for the greater good; it's all about the message not the messenger.

By the end of the first day I was on cloud nine; I knew that my persistence had paid off, lomilomi was truly my missing link and the last piece of the jigsaw. It would still take a few more years before the stardance was completed and ready to rain down on the peoples of the world, but for now I knew that the 40-year quest was about to finish and the responsibility to share was about to start. I was bursting at the seams and wanted to tell everyone but could not. Before that could happen, I needed to check in with the guardians, the keepers of the secret; this was not about my wants, my needs, or my ego!!

Many thanks, Tom, your workshop was inspirational.

Some time after this experience, a kahuna said to me that it is a Hawaiian tradition for the student to ask three times before being granted his wish; the workshop in St. Pete's had been my third attempt at finding lomilomi. Now I find out that it was never lomilomi on trial, it was me who was on trial, I was being tested by the very entities that I was working with... the last laugh was truly on me!

1:8 Aloha

A hello or goodbye,
An acknowledgement, a look in the eye.
A smile, kind gesture or communication,
A loving attempt to make a connection.
Gentleness, patience and caring,
Honor, respect and sharing.

Creating a positive attitude,
Living and being in gratitude.
A handshake, hug or a kiss,
Love yourself and extend the bliss.
Share the rainbow of your heart,
And you will become a part,
Of a circle with no ending or start.

A wave of aloha rolling in and out,
While never having a second thought or doubt,
Of what life is really all about.
In the Spirit of Aloha.

Tina Marie Fair

"Great spirits have always encountered violent opposition from mediocre minds."

Albert Einstein

1:9 Dyslexia

This is a subject that I have had to deal with all my life; however, only a handful of people know that this is a condition I have to deal with. (Notice I don't refer to it as a condition that affects me. It doesn't, I deal with it.)

Dyslexia comes in a number of guises and my story may not be that of others; however, if it helps just one person to take control of the condition and improve their lives, my 'coming out' will have been worth it.

There are many reasons for keeping it quiet and most are based on survival in what can be a hard world, especially if you are perceived as being different or less intelligent, simply because it takes time to 'interpret the language' being used. The same misconception is often applied to people with a stammer; they speak slower and are wrongly perceived as being slower. I understood how the world worked at a young age, it's all about perception. So once I left school and all my school mates behind, they knew my difficulty. I put in place all sorts of coping mechanisms in order to deal with the problem and my biggest fear was to be found out; I feared the loss of respect and a repeat of the humiliation I had faced in my school years. Nowadays I am comfortable in my own skin, don't have to prove anything to anybody, and more importantly, don't care what others might say or think about me or this condition.

The other reason I have kept it quiet for so long is that it has become quite fashionable to be dyslexic. There are many celebrities claiming to have been affected by it, the condition is often used as a marketing tool in much the same way as some celebrities use the unsubstantiated claim of child abuse for the sympathy vote. Other times the condition is being used as an excuse for not achieving: 'I've got dyslexia so I will never be able to do that'. This may have worked for some, but I used it as a lifetime motivational tool, I was going to prove my teacher and my class mates wrong.

What is dyslexia? Dyslexia or word blindness was first identified in 1881 by Oswald Berkhan, but it was not until the 1970s with a new hypothesis that dyslexia stems from a deficit in phonological processing that the condition was taken seriously. Further studies in 1979 by Galburda and Kemper and autopsy examinations in 1985 by Galburda observed anatomical differences in the language center in a dyslexic brain. A bridge of tissue in the middle of the brain called the corpus callosum is out of whack. Reading material that should go to the left side of the brain goes to the right side as well and the two sides are out of sync.

Dyslexia is a severe language problem of neurological origin in a person with average or above average intelligence for whom there are no other physical, medical or psychological conditions sufficiently serious to account for language handling deficits. These findings helped the establishment to accept dyslexia and to set up educational studies and teaching strategies.

The left side of the brain can match a letter with its sound, handle information in strings, like the sounds in a word, one letter after another, rather than seeing a word as a single picture. It can also understand grammar and syntax. The right side is different. It deals in areas of space and patterns. It doesn't understand parts of speech, or keep track of letter order in spelling. It 'reads' a word as a line drawing that it has been taught has a meaning, a single sketch (which can be a drawing or a word) and not a line-up of sounds.

However, dyslexic people are highly creative, intuitive, and excel at three-dimensional problem solving and hands-on learning. Their visual and holistic learning style means that they learn best through the creative process, with methods that focus on mastery of the meanings of words and symbols. When learning methods that fit the thinking style are used, dyslexics can excel in academics and read and write efficiently. The true gift of dyslexia is the gift of mastery.

Looking back

I now see that all the evidence was there, but the 'D' word did not exist when I was young. It was replaced by other 'D' words such as Dunce, Dopy, Dippy, Daft, and Dimwit or simply just Dumb. I was a late developer at school; my early years were spent in a South London Victorian-built inner city school where, if you struggled with reading and writing, you were simply left behind and treated as stupid. In a recent conversation with my now 80 year-old mother, she revealed that she was so worried about my slow development in reading that she took me to the local doctor, who simply told her to buy books that I was interested in. But I was not interested in any books because I could not read the words, so she bought me a comic and I entered a world of wonder. You see, I see words phonically and why is the word phonically not spelt phonically? I pronounce words as I see them and spell them as I say them, which is OK until you have to deal with the English language which includes words that have silent letters, and different ways of pronouncing words based on your geographical location. I often had frustrating lessons with my English teacher until I discovered the rule of the secret 'R'. You see, in London, if you take a word like tomato it is pronounced as 'tom mar toe' so when I was asked to spell tomato I would spell it 'tom mar to' and include the 'R' sound that my teacher made. The response from the teacher, as he raised his voice, would go something like this: "No, you stupid boy, break it down, it's TOM MAR TOE"...

We would go round in circles; often I was left thinking 'what is it that I cannot see, what don't I understand?' and this same rule applied to other words like bath which is pronounced in London as barth. It was much later before I was exposed to other dialects (we had limited TV in those days and only the public school BBC type of language was used). It was a revelation to hear a northerner saying bath, or an American saying tomato. This was when I realized that I was not stupid. My rationale was that it was the teachers who did not or could not recognize the problem they had; my problem was not a language one, but simply one of location.

With this insight I was able to develop another language; my own translation language was an effective strategy that would help me through my school days and beyond. The rule of the secret 'R' was implemented with great success. However, it did rely on experience and memory. I would often trip up when I came across a word that was new to me, one that I did not have in the memory bank; however, once I had visualized it and added it to my new language, I was OK. This was to become the first of many survival mechanisms implemented throughout my life to deal with what was then an unknown problem. I was intuitively developing new learning methods that fitted in with my thinking style.

Another example of a simple word that caused the biggest problems would be the word 'does'. You see, a lot of dyslexics use visualization as a thinking model. The word 'doe' is a female deer, so logically two or more female deer would be 'does', but somehow in the English language when you add 's' to the word 'doe', the sound of the 'o' changes to the sound of a 'u' – this was very confusing to a schoolboy struggling with the English language. In order to overcome this, I would first have to visualize the word 'does' then change it into its visual translation word of 'dus' in order to pronounce it.

School days

I had mixed feelings at high school and mixed experiences, but I never missed a day. I loved sports, art, drama, woodwork and any hands-on activity; I loved 'doing things' but struggled with math and English and endured a daily humiliation by way of a verbal math or spelling test. For the first three years in high school we had a teacher – who I shall call Mr White – who would finish the day by making the whole class stand up and then ask each child in turn to spell a chosen word. When they got it right they could sit down and only when everyone was seated could the class go home.

This would result in the same five pupils standing at the end of each day enduring a barrage of 'D' words (see above) from the teacher, and moans and groans and even threats from the other class mates. As the pressure increased, so did the reality of finding the correct spelling. The effect of this was frustration, feelings of inferiority and poor self-esteem. But I would experience the opposite when involved in sport and would often use this medium as a 'payback' for the classroom bullies.

Two of this group of five combated their frustrations and daily humiliation by playing up, being disruptive and even walking out of class. They would rather get detention or go on report then face the daily abuse. One pupil started to miss the last lesson of the day on the pretence of religious commitments and he eventually changed schools. All of these were survival strategies and I needed one of my own. You may well ask why was it we didn't say anything. But you see, to us this way of teaching was normal; we had no way of knowing that other teachers taught any differently. Also when you have dyslexia it can make it difficult to express yourself clearly using vocabulary and to structure thoughts during a conversation.

After the first year I became aware that the teacher would repeat various words often in blocks of three or four. I set myself a task of learning these blocks by repetition. Then as the number of students standing was reduced by getting the spelling right, I knew that sooner or later the teacher would start on one of these blocks of words, and if that was two or three students further down the line from me, I would know in advance which word I was going to get and had time to visualize it before being asked to spell it.

It worked a treat – eventually I would always be seated about halfway through the daily testing process. The downside was that my teacher thought the methods worked and I never did (at least during my school days) learn the other 100 or so words.

Motivation

My motivation for life's challenges could always be found subconsciously in the words of my school teacher: Dunce, Dopy, Dippy, Daft, and Dimwit and my response would be: I'll show him...

After finishing school I started to excel in various areas of my life: business, education, sport, and family, gradually achieving one life goal after another. I came to realize that I was using a negative experience to prove that I was good enough and not stupid. But who was I proving this to? The teacher was no longer a part of my life, or at least not in person; was I trying to prove it to a memory? Was I trying to prove it to myself as part of my self-esteem? I was about to find out on a NLP practitioner's course.

Acceptance

Acceptance of dyslexia would allow me the freedom of expression and the carefree enlightenment of a quantum leap of understanding. I have often followed my 'gut feelings' when booking courses and workshops, and this was no different. I had read about and studied Huna for a number of years and this led to a study of the mind which inevitably included neuro-linguistic programming (NLP). I had found a practitioner's course on the South Coast of England that included hypnotherapy and Timeline therapy. I had no intention of becoming a NLP practitioner but the course content was of value to me; I also thought it was time to deal with the dyslexia question.

When I first heard about dyslexia in the 1980s, I was pleased that they had found a real 'something' – at last I had an answer to my many questions and why my many coping strategies worked.

Even though I had come to realise that this was the problem, it would be many years before I would accept and admit this to the world. At the time, dyslexia was being used by a lot of people as an excuse for failure. I was not a failure, I was motivated in life and my strategies were successful – why change them? I had internal acceptance and understanding, so why share this with the world, I reasoned.

Now I realise that the life I've enjoyed is the very reason to share my story with the world; if it helps just one person I will be happy. I have an absolute belief that anyone can do anything if they dedicate the time and effort required to achieve it – something I have proved to myself time and time again. If I can do it with an undiagnosed condition then others, with the advantages of modern science and education, can also achieve their dreams.

Now was the time to put my ghost to bed, and in order to do that I needed to make a public acceptance about the fact that I was dyslexic. The course was to help in my understanding of how the mind works and how the brain interprets the information it receives.

NLP has a process called anchoring during which you can associate an emotional state with a physical action. For example, if you feel happy, very happy, and at the height of that stimulus you touched your index finger, then if every time you reached that happiness high or you remember a period when you were that happy you also touched your index finger, you will create an anchor. After a while you should be able to touch your index finger and bring on the feelings of happiness.

I can achieve feelings of motivation by recycling the old negative school experience and the desire to 'show him', thus building an anchor on a negative emotion. I needed to revisit those bad days in order to move forward and build a future on a positive anchor. The opportunity arose during a Timeline therapy session. My student partner took me back in time, way back to those schoolboy days. I experienced what I had experienced, I felt what I had felt – the pain, the humiliation, the sadness. I had tears in my eyes as I watched my schoolboy self in front of that class. I was able to reach out and help, to reassure him that everything will be all right, the future will take care of itself and in doing so I was able to change the past. The very fact that I am writing this book illustrates that you can face and overcome your demons. If I can do it, and I am no better than you, then believe me you can do it too.

Shamanic Dream

That night I slept like a baby, a deep restful sleep until the early hours, and then I slid into a shamanic dream, a parallel universe, where things are not quite what they seem. I knew what was happening as I had had similar experiences before. I was drifting through cloud-like structures when I heard the spirit of my old teacher. I could just make out some of his facial features, with soft wispy outlines; there was an air of sadness about the vision. I had a feeling that he wanted to give me a gift, a gift of knowledge, and with that came a knowing, a knowing of how my mind worked, how my mind processed information. This was passed over to me in a clear vision, as clear as watching TV in high definition. I could see snippets of information energy enter my mind, how I made choices as to which piece of information to keep for later use, which piece to act on immediately and which to let go. I could see how these choices could be influenced by beliefs and upbringing; I could see the chemical interchange in the body and the emotional release that followed; I was shown how to change this linked reaction on an emotional, chemical, intellectual and physical basis.

I was then shown how my mind processed information to overcome the so-called dyslexia problem, how information was turned into vision, and how vision was used as a translation medium to overcome written and verbal language interaction. I was informed that we dyslexics were pioneers; we were wired for the future when all communication from human to human and human to animal would simply be a telegraphic visual thought experience. We were here so that the human race can take the next step and learn about the unlimited power of the mind and move towards a time when communication will no longer be limited to a collection of agreed vocal grunts. Visual communication through thought process is a futuristic advanced form of communication seen by a world not yet ready for it. It's a bit like introducing a Smart interactive TV to a world that can only communicate through Morse code; blind in their ignorance, they say communicate in the way that we do or you must be stupid. It's like putting a Chinese-speaking child into an English-speaking class and expecting him to respond at the same level and at the same speed as the other children. Are they any less intelligent than the other children because they don't communicate in the same language? Dunce, Dopy, Dippy, Daft, Dimwit – now when I hear this, I don't feel angry, hurt, upset or sad for I know what they have yet to know, and I have seen what they have yet to see.

Forgiveness

After the technicolor vision had finished, I had an overwhelming sense of oneness and gratitude. I had a knowing that the spirit teacher I had just seen had my best interests at heart and wanted forgiveness for a lack of knowledge during his embodiment. A great sadness came over me as I realized that I had entrapped part of his spirit and I had used it as a negative motivational force for my own needs. It was I who needed to ask for forgiveness and to release his spirit to go on its way. What followed was a starburst moment, one of complete love and happiness, one that happens when we are in alignment with the power of the universe, leaving a radiant glow of gratitude which led me back into a deep sleep.

The next day I shared the experience with the other students on the course and now I share it with you...

The Dyslexic Brain

I must emphasize that this model was given to me about how my brain processes information; it may or may not apply to you. If it helps just one person then this chapter is worth its inclusion in this book.

The brain works like any central communication center and can be divided into five working parts:

1 **Control Center**

2 **The Big Screen**

3 **Translation Center**

4 **Quick Reference Guide (for emergency use)**

5 **Panic Button**

1 *Control Center*

All information from all of the senses comes into my control center where it is distributed directly to its relevant area. Often we respond through knowledge, through habit and by way of the unconscious mind. However, in this example we are going to follow the action after the control center is verbally presented with a word that needs the action of the conscious mind in order to spell it.

2 *The Big Screen*

The word is first flashed up on to the big screen; at this point we will often pull information straight from the memory banks and spell the word correctly on the big screen. That information is then passed on by the vocal cords to the outside world.

However, if the word is not spelt phonetically or cannot be pulled up from the memory banks, only part of the word will appear on the big screen; this will trigger the next action.

3 *Translation Center*

The word is sent to the translation center where we look into the files of our advanced translation language and check for things like a secret 'R' or a silent 'P' or any other rule or device to translate the incoming sound (of the word) into a word that we can spell. The sound TOM MAR TOE is hence changed into TOMATO by using the American pronunciation which is phonetically correct. This word can then be flashed up on to the big screen, so that it can be visualized and then passed on by the vocal cords to the outside world, spelt correctly.

All this assumes that we have time and are not under any pressure to produce a result.

However, if the translation center is under pressure from external stress, this can produce misfiring of the electrical circuit with the wrong partner word popping on to the screen. Resulting in a genuine misspelling, you spell the word that you can see correctly, but it's not the word that you were asked to spell.

If the translation center is put under pressure while searching for a word during a conversation, it may cause you to abandon the translation center in favor of the quick reference guide.

4 *Quick Reference Guide*

Is a bit of a cop-out, but it gives you an alternative word very quickly and allows you to deflect any possible awkwardness; it's basically a get-out-of-jail card. The downside is the alternative word may only consist of one or two syllables and you may appear to have a limited vocabulary if it is used too often. The other problem is that due to outside pressure, once this replacement word is found it will be expressed forward, bypassing all checks of translation and acceptance. (Some people's QRG is full of swear words and not appropriate in most situations.)

5 *Survival Button*

Often referred to as the panic button and will trigger the primal survival response of fight, flight or freeze. This is often seen in children when all of the above has failed or if they are under pressure from a teacher. The response is to throw a tantrum (fight) or run out of the class (flight) or go into their shell, sulk, or have a moody (freeze).

The future

Writing this book has been great therapy; it has been a way of proving to me (yet again) that I can overcome all obstacles, in this case dyslexia. Hopefully it will be helpful or even inspirational to others. For further reading go to dyslexia.com

People who are crazy enough to think that they can change the world are the ones who do.

Apple Computers

1:10 Don't tell me what I can't do

Just like everyone else, my self-esteem had its ups and downs during my childhood and teenage years. I was in my element while playing sport, managing football teams, being a Boy Scout patrol leader – even taking responsibility for the safety and upbringing of my brother and sisters all added to my self-esteem. And then came school, my undiagnosed and unrecognized condition of dyslexia, and the daily humiliation that accompanied it.

I have a very good West Indian friend who had a similar experience, but in his case it was race related. I met Desmond shortly after he arrived in this country from the West Indies in the early sixties. He has a larger than life personality, full of energy, and a loving mum who, if anything, has a personality even larger than Desmond's. As street kids we both loved football. Desmond joined my group of friends and fitted in immediately, he was just another one of us, no more and certainly no less. Even though our life was hard, we enjoyed it and went everywhere together.

And then one day at school, it happened!

Just like me, Desmond struggled with the teaching of the English language. Looking back I can see that Desmond's hyperactive nature had all the symptoms of Attention Deficit Disorder (ADD).

Because they didn't understand dyslexia, I was branded as slow, even a troublemaker, because my concentration levels fluctuated and my attention wandered. Desmond had to put up with similar problems; however, on this particular day it was pointed out to us by the teacher that it was not his fault, it was because he, you guessed it... was black.

You know, until that moment I didn't even realize that he was black. In our group of friends we had blond hair, brown hair, black hair and red hair. We had white skin, coffee-colored skin and black skin; we even had one lad with freckly skin that would go bright red in the summer. But these colors and other identifying features are just a part of who we are, but never, ever, did it define us.

We both had just received a lesson in life: for the first time we were being told that we were different, and that we were in some way a lesser person because of those differences. We were constantly being told that we would amount to nothing. We were being mentally separated from the other boys and went through a process of daily humiliation. This eventually erodes your self-esteem and if you let it, you will reach a point where you feel worthless, or you rebel. We both rebelled, but we were left with a lifetime's desire to prove ourselves.

'Don't tell me what I can't do' had become our motto.

I think we both spent many years hunting for that lost self-esteem from our school days. One way we have done this is through qualifications and titles, always putting ourselves to the test in order to prove that we are good enough. Desmond gained a law degree and is now a successful businessman. I started collecting initials after my name; after all, I reasoned to myself, the world could then see that I was as good as them. I became a letter junkie, first behind my name and then in front of my name.

I learned from this process that anyone can achieve anything if they are willing to pay the price. The price is often high, in time and commitment, but when you truly set out to achieve something, put your mind to it, backed up by 100% effort, there is nothing that can stop you.

If you want titles and qualifications, I wish you good fortune, but make sure that you are doing it for the right reasons.

I can honestly say that these days there are only two titles that bring a smile to my face: husband and dad. Sorry, there are now three – and 'granddad'!

> *"Love your life, perfect your life, beautify all things in your life..."*
>
> Tecumseh

1:11 A Cherokee Legend

An old Cherokee is teaching his grandson about life. "A fight is going on inside me," he said to the boy.

The old grandfather said to his grandson, who came to him with anger at a friend who had done him an injustice, "Let me tell you a story. I too, at times, have felt a great hate for those that have taken so much, with no sorrow for what they do.

But hate wears you down, and does not hurt your enemy. It is like taking poison and wishing your enemy would die. I have struggled with these feelings many times." He continued, "It is as if there are two wolves inside me engaged in a terrible fight.

One is evil – he is anger, envy, sorrow, regret, greed, arrogance, self-pity, guilt, resentment, inferiority, lies, false pride, superiority, and ego. The littlest thing will set him into a fit of temper. He fights everyone, all the time, for no reason. He cannot think because his anger and hate are so great. It is helpless anger, for his anger will change nothing.

But the other wolf, ah! He is good and does no harm. He is joy, peace, love, hope, serenity, humility, kindness, benevolence, empathy, generosity, truth, compassion, and faith. The same fight is going on inside you – and inside every other person, too.

He lives in harmony with all around him, and does not take offense when no offense was intended. He will only fight when it is right to do so, and in the right way.

Sometimes, it is hard to live with these two wolves inside me, for both of them try to dominate my spirit."

The boy thought about it for a minute, looked intently into his grandfather's eyes and asked, "Which wolf will win, Grandfather?"

The grandfather smiled and quietly said: "The one I feed."

He who seeks revenge should first dig two graves...

Confucius

1:12 Forgiveness

"I am not being told to forgive my enemies, I am not made that way, I do feel resentment against them, and therefore I am not going to read this section." This is a common response to the word forgiveness.

Why do we respond, often quite forcibly, to the suggestion that we should forgive those who have wronged us? I have come to realize that religious leaders advocate but often do not practice unconditional forgiveness, and as non-perfect humans it is a standard that is quite beyond most of us. It may be something that we acknowledge subconsciously and reject consciously. Afraid of being reminded of our non-perfect status, we simply bypass any chapter referring to forgiveness.

I, too, struggled with this for many years, and as a result life kept re-presenting the lesson in different formats until I eventually 'took the bull by the horns' and faced up to the reality of non-forgiveness. Forgiveness and non-forgiveness are simply the two wolves referred to by the Cherokee grandfather and only the one you feed will survive.

For me, the secret of forgiveness was to turn it on its head and start with non-forgiveness and its effects on one's self. The effect is not only an emotional/chemical one 'the brain is a pharmacy' but also a disempowering one.

When we are angry because someone has trespassed against us (done something to upset us) we produce hormones and chemicals that will support the feeling of anger. Through neurotransmitters, emotions follow thought and negative emotions release an onslaught of damaging chemicals with the consequent effect on our immune system. The brain's pharmacy is the pituitary gland and is controlled by the hypothalamus. These operate a number of glands through the endocrine system that secrete various hormones into the bloodstream. A constant state of stress caused by the chemicals of negative thinking will eventually take its toll on our health.

Get this straight: energy follows thought, thought results in emotion, emotion leads to chemical/hormonal release into the bloodstream. You are literally poisoning yourself with negative, fearful, depressing or angry thoughts. No one else is doing this to you – it's self-inflicted!

If we continue to replay the scenario again and again over many years, we build on the anger and resentment and slowly poison ourselves with negative energy and emotion. Each time we do this we thicken the energy cord that keeps us attached to the perpetrator and in doing so we make them a permanent and prominent part of our lives. We are simply handing over power to that person.

That person or that event may have hit you hard; learn from it but don't let it define you. You need to take back your power, take responsibility for your response to the person or event. You may not have been able to stop it happening in the first place, but you do have a choice: you let them keep the power they have stolen from you or you take it back.

Conditional forgiveness

This is a formula, a practical step that works for those non-perfect humans among us. Let the self-righteous religious leaders keep their demand for unconditional forgiveness; I for one find it unpractical for use at my level of spiritual growth, I am still working towards unconditional love and forgiveness. Conditional forgiveness, however, works for me; it allows me to take a step in the right direction, improves my health, removes any hold the perpetrator believes he or she has, and lets me take back the power without hurting anyone.

What is conditional forgiveness and how does it work? Well, first you have to get to a place where forgiveness is possible.

Many years ago I was betrayed by someone that I regarded as a good friend. At the time, I had a young family and was working all hours to pay the mortgage and the bills. Life was a struggle and we had little savings. But we were a happy family, we appreciated and enjoyed the little things in life, we always made time for our children and would take them away somewhere on vacation most years. Because we concentrated on the good things, we must have given the impression that life was OK. Unbeknown to us at the time, our family happiness caused jealousy and resentment in those who did not appreciate what they had, which in material terms was a lot more than us.

We were very good friends with another couple who also had two children and we even had a holiday or two together. When the husband was made redundant from a computer servicing company, he proposed that we invest our small amount of savings into his new business as a competitor computer servicing company. This business was to be sustained by various companies who were loyal to our friend and letters of pending contracts seemed to support his proposal. However, as it would require all our savings, we hesitated and delayed our decision over a number of months. Eventually, I backed up my wife who was in turn supporting her relationship with her close friend, the wife of our potential business partner.

As with all new businesses, the first year was hard, and so it proved, but we had monthly reports that suggested not only was our money safe, but long term would prove to be a wise investment. What we did not know or find out until the end of the financial year was the fact that our 'friend' did not obtain a single contract of service from any of his 'loyal' contacts, all the monthly reports he had produced were fictitious and his so-called contract meetings were in fact job interviews for himself. He ended up being employed by a large bank and we lost all our savings and nearly our home.

Now this is someone who does not deserve forgiveness was my response. I was to fester on the betrayal for a number of years: how could someone I called a friend, someone I trusted, treat us like that? Resentment grew and also my level of anger every time I thought about the situation. To make things worse, what followed for us was several years of financial hardship, while he had all the trappings of a large income. Life did not appear fair.

Then one day after attending a Huna workshop, I realized that those eight to twelve months of betrayal had turned into eight years of resentment and I was feeding energy into the resentment fire, keeping it alive, while I waited for an apology that was unlikely to ever arrive.

I no longer wanted this person to be a part of my life; he had taken a lot from me in terms of money and trust. But I had given him more in terms of life energy and now I was unwilling to feed this parasite any longer. The question was how to free myself from him without letting him off the hook; it's that non-perfect human in me again. The answer was to be found in a shamanic experience that I termed as conditional forgiveness.

Step 1 - *first you need to get to a place where forgiveness is possible. Ask yourself what would need to happen for you to be able to forgive, no matter how implausible that might be. We are not looking for reality, we are looking for possibility.*

Most of us want recognition that we have been wronged, followed by a sincere request for forgiveness.

Some of you may want punishment – that's fine at this stage, we are simply trying to get to a place (after a number of conditions have been met) where you find that you could forgive the trespass against you.

Step 2 - *once you have arrived and accepted that forgiveness is possible (subject to conditions) I want you to feel the emotion of forgiveness. Don't forget we are now in a place where all of your conditions have been met, so really feel the emotion of forgiving, feel the emotional release of being told that you are right and were wronged. Feel the power of being asked to forgive the perpetrator who with all their heart wants your blessing.*

Now capture this emotion and place it in a small helium-filled balloon, tie it with a very fine, unbreakable thread of light and connect it to the shoulder of the person you are willing to forgive (if they request it).

Ask for forgiveness from them for any wrong, either real or perceived, that they feel you have done – this may even be feeding the fire of resentment. When you have done this you will feel a lot lighter.

This person now has your full forgiveness attached to them for life; all they have to do is request forgiveness from you, even if it's on their death bed. They just have to ask with sincerity and they will receive it. You, in turn, have requested forgiveness from them for any wrongs, real or perceived, against them. This is important as we all have a different view of reality; you are not giving them any power, just simply 'wiping the slate clean' for after this exercise there will be no future contact, either physical or energetic.

Some say that with unconditional forgiveness you are trying to force your will (of forgiveness) on to someone who may not want it, or may even violently refuse it. You don't have that right. With conditional forgiveness you are providing the means by which forgiveness can happen, and in doing so severing your contact. But you are also allowing for the spiritual growth of the other entity; rest assured they will at some time – during this life or the next – request the forgiveness you have graciously prepared.

Step 3 - the final step is to sever the energy attachment to this person; in Huna these energy cords are called 'Aka cords'. The more energy you have sent down the cord (positive or negative), the thicker the cord and your connection to that person will be.

Imagine an intense bright light above your head, breathe in the light, deep into your stomach, and fill your body with each breath. Once you have this bright light energy in every part of your body, put a silk tourniquet around the cord at your end and cut the cord so no energy can ever return. Now, with a deep out breath, release a generous blast of light down the cord (just like dragon's fire-breath), watch it burn and consume the cord, starting at your end and traveling all the way down until it is detached and gone. Breathe more light energy into yourself and replace the energy that was used to burn the cord. If the cord was thick and the connection very strong you may need to repeat the ritual whenever you feel a possible re-growth; once or twice is usually enough to cut the other person completely out of your life.

If you feel vulnerable, breathe out and surround yourself with a protective firewall; this will burn up and destroy any attempt of *reattachment from the other person. Wish them well and let them go on their way, complete with your forgiveness balloon.*

Summary *– you can't be angry and hateful and at the same time be in a state of love and bliss.*

You may not be able to stop people hurting you, but you do have a choice as to how long you will allow that hurt to survive. Why would you swap one moment of love and happiness for the fire of hate and anger?

Remember you are not hurting the person who has wronged you, you are only hurting yourself. Don't give them that power!

> *"When you hold resentment toward another, you are bound to that person or condition by an emotional link that is stronger than steel. Forgiveness is the only way to dissolve that link and get free."*
>
> Catherine Ponder

Forgive ourselves

And finally – when we forgive others, who are we forgiving? We are forgiving ourselves, of course. Do you want to be right or do you want to be happy?

Learning to forgive yourself is a great start. Forgive yourself for any bad thought towards others, it's just a thought and through chemical reaction you are the one that suffered. The same applies to anger, frustration or any other negative thought or action. Your emotional computer is working within the limitations of the human form, you are not your body or your mind, and you are spirit embodied.

Open yourself to forgiveness, find a quiet spot, relax and take a deep breath in through your nose while focusing on your stomach, then let it out through your mouth while focusing on your heart.

As you continue to breathe, switch your attention to your inner spirit, your unhuman soul, then with all your heart say: "I am sorry, I love you, please forgive me." Repeat this until you come to a place of acceptance. Then take another breath, focus on your heart and the love of aloha, now say: "I forgive me, for my reaction to the experience and I promise to approach it in a different way should the experience ever be repeated, thank you, I love you." Take a deep breath and say: "It is done... Mahalo and blessings." Experience that the incident or feeling has been forgiven and the wish has flown back to the heavens.

You can expand on this by having a list of specific things that you want to forgive yourself for, go back in time as far as needed, forgiving and releasing as you go. Feel the pain, the hurt, the shame, see it without judgement, thank it for the experience, say: "Thank you, please forgive me" (for my reaction); with your focus on your inner spirit say: "I love you."

This is the first step towards the quantum leap of unconditional forgiveness, learning to love and to forgive yourself.

Remember, one baby step at a time...

The time of prophesy is now.

The secrets are simple and often right in front of your face.

1:13 Is there a God?

My mother is ambidextrous – she is naturally left-handed but with the help of the sisters at her convent school she learned to write with both hands. This help came in the form of a sharp whack across the knuckles with a wooden ruler if she committed the sin of writing with her left hand. Apparently, her soul has also been commended to an eternity of hot fires

because she married my father who was not a Catholic. She is not perturbed by this, and would say: "I hate the cold, and the heat will be good for my arthritis."

Apparently, even after she was married the priest would knock on her door, ranting and raving about her sinful actions. My mother and father were married for over 40 years before being separated by death. They had four children, nine grandchildren, and three great-grandchildren; I ask you, how can that be wrong?

As bad as it was I must admit to being grateful, for out of that experience came a new attitude to religion. My parents had a strict Victorian upbringing that was founded on the church – Catholic and Anglican. They believed in right and wrong and considered a foundation based on these principles was good for their offspring, but they were against any strict or extreme religious teaching. Therefore, in our formative years we were to attend Sunday school but would have the freedom of choice once we reached an age of responsibility.

My childhood experience of God and the bible was quite confusing. At Sunday school I learned about Jesus and all the good he did, but when I was introduced to the bible, and we started with the Old Testament, I found that Jesus was the son of a fearful, vengeful God. God is love said the bible, but he will also take your life away and condemn you to hell if you dare cross him.

At the age of ten I made one of my biggest life-changing decisions. I loved Jesus, or at least the spirit of love and kindness that he stood for, but I could not support this tyrant of a father. I was in conflict with myself. How could I possibly have thoughts that went against my upbringing? At that time in the 1960s you were either religious or an atheist; I wanted to be neither of these and decided at this very young age to love and follow the spirit of Jesus but reject the tyrant that was God. It was the first step on a new path, a path we now refer to as a 'spiritual pathway'.

Nowadays, I seldom use the word God as it has so many confusing connotations. I prefer terms such as higher power, the universe, the force, the light, the spirit of aloha, or simply spirit – I use these terms interchangeably. When I talk about spirit, I am referring to the spirit of aloha, which in turn is the spirit of love, the Divine. If any of these terms are not particularly meaningful to you, please feel free to substitute them with whatever word you prefer. You can even choose the word God.

This new path gave me the freedom to explore other religions and beliefs. It was to take me through the doors of churches, mosques, synagogues and temples around the world. Many would talk about love, but not many would walk their talk. More people have been killed because of religion than for any other reason. If God is love then why don't those who choose to follow him have any tolerance for others? Many of those in charge of religions seem to seek to control the behavior of their devotees, and even use them to try and change the behavior of followers of other religions. This isn't the action of love; it's the action of ego and power. I have seen much good in all peoples of the earth, but I have also seen the darkness that descends when people live in fear – fear of others or even their own God.

The one thing that remained constant and kept me company on this path of discovery was the spirit of Jesus, the universal spirit of love. I traveled this path always looking for answers, for information. I have had doubts, fears and hardship, but I always knew that the pathway was heading in the right direction.

This path would eventually lead me back to the oldest spiritual way known to man – shamanism – and eventually to the spirit of aloha. The spirit of aloha is the spirit of love, and love is the foundation of all religions.

I have arrived at a place of complete trust in the higher power of the universe that is found within me and within everyone and everything that exists.

Every now and then, when the universe thinks I am ready, it will once again reveal another of its secrets. One of these gems of knowledge brought God back into my life, but in a completely new form; as Spock once said in Star Trek: "There's life, Jim, but not as we know it." I was sitting in traffic on a cold winter's morning, high on a hill in Crystal Palace, a suburb of South London, when I saw a sign outside a church which read 'God is love'. I have seen this sign many times before. It was the same message taken from the bible in my childhood days, which I have always taken as meaning that this person, this powerful figure, this entirety that we call God is not only the creator, the power of the universe, the judge 'on judgement day' the jury 'passing judgement' but he was also now love. I have rejected this message as a contradiction on many occasions.

However, today was different. As I looked at the sign, the words seemed to move, it was as though I was decoding the message in order to find the hidden truth. And there it was − it no longer read 'God is love'. The message was clear, it was simple, and how could I have not seen it before?

The words 'LOVE IS GOD' stood before me, the universe had just revealed one of its gems, an ultimate truth.

For me, this simple knowing changed everything: the power of the universe did not belong to the 'old man in the sky'. The power of the universe is the divine energy of love, which for oceanic people is the spirit of aloha. This is my truth, my viewpoint from where I stand on the pathway to the stars, somewhere on the mountain of knowledge. It may not be your view from where you stand, and that is also OK.

Anyone who has experienced a moment of true love, a moment when the power of love gave us the greatest feeling of our lives, when love gave us the power to face our greatest fear or even the willingness to surrender life itself for the benefit of another, knows deep down in their soul the truth of this statement.

At this point we need to explore the word love, for I know that many have trouble with this concept. Most of the problems stem from a western upbringing and education system – a system that leads us to believe that there is only one word for love and that is love. A thought process that leads us to think you are either in love, or not in love. The good book states that you should love thy neighbor. You may say that I love my wife, my husband, my children, even my dog, I might even like my neighbor but I can't love them because it would in some way devalue the love I have for my family.

From an oceanic point of view, love can be used like a bowl of sugar. If you add a little sugar you can make things sweeter. If you add too much you can overpower the experience. The art is in applying the right amount in the right situation. For that, we need degrees or a measure, with sugar it's grains or spoonfuls. With love it's words such as caring, kindness, affection, helpful, considerate, thoughtful, compassion, mercy, sympathy, liking, honest, honor, truthful. Each one of these words has a few gains or the 'essence of love' in them, some more than others. The art is in choosing the right word or the right action to match the appropriate situation. You can see now that by expanding the meaning of the word love we can indeed love thy neighbor by 'liking thy neighbor' or 'helping thy neighbor'. Each one of these words uses a few grains of love energy, or if applied to action, as in helping them, you are actively using the power of the universe.

It was the aloha spirit that helped me understand the true essence of love, and in that quantum leap the universe revealed yet another gem.

The energy source that is complete unconditional love is the Divine, the source of all. Remember 'Love is God' – it's the source of universal energy. The word love carries many elements, each defining the amount of love energy found in the action it pertains to. The ultimate word for love energy is grace, meaning energy from divine love, or love from the divine source. Grace is the empowering presence of love energy.

We can therefore refer to this energy of unconditional love from the divine source as Grace of Divinity or GOD – love truly is God.

In many ancient cultures, the universe is represented by the symbol 'O' and if you add that 'O' to the English word god, you have 'good'. To be here and to do 'good' work in the face of adversity is to be working in grace with the energy of the Divine.

As Spock said in Star Trek: "There is a God, Jim, but not as we know him!"

The Source:

Ku, God, Jehovah, Allah, Inner Light, Love – one eternal truth.

What does a great power care what we call him? Little minds put tags on things and people; love accepts and encompasses all matter and all beings. Humans have been given the right to make choices: to be good or evil, to be gods or stones.

We are all born with that perfect power to do and be all things. We have the right to do with it whatever we wish. If we keep our bowl free from rocks, we can go forward and backward in time, walk with the angels, climb the heights and live in paradise.

> *"It is everyone's own decision where and what he is."*
>
> Ka Hopena

"It has been my direct experience that what most westerners think of as the father (or mother) is actually a beginning-less and endless field of light that some know as the source or Yao, a vast sea of timeless energy that is charged with potential. And this luminous source is everywhere because everything is a manifestation of it.

This discovery in turn brings the seeker into direct experience of the field of magnified power that underlies and infuses

everything everywhere with life force... a field of which your
own soul is a part... that same field that many call God."

- Hank Wesselman

Spirit beings

We are more real than our present reality, more solid and more spirit than outer circumstances reflect. The body is a communication tool, a home, a vessel for travel and entertainment of spirit while on this physical planet. In short, we are spirit beings here to have a human experience. Here is another gem of universal truth – we are immortal spiritual beings who exist separately from our bodies.

"The spirit of man is not evil in his soul, he is divine in his soul, for his soul comes from the source of all that is, the divine power. We are spirit beings, we come from the source of all, we are energy seeds of love, we need to grow and to grow we need to experience that which we are not.

How can you really love if you have not experienced hate? How can you heal if you have not experienced suffering? How can you know joy if you don't know hurt? This is the reason we are here, these are the lessons we must learn. We are here to experience the dark side, experience an opposite way of living, that's why to 'live' in reverse is called 'evil' and to have 'lived' in reverse is to have spent time with the 'devil'. There is no horned beast to tempt us, in the cosmic make-up of all that is there is no such thing as evil. We are here to experience everything that is, is there anything humans have not done to each other? We are here to witness and experience life here on earth. Our challenge is to try and change the way of the physical dimension by the application of love.

If you choose to believe there is good and evil, then that is your truth, and you are not wrong at all. But, remember, it is your truth; it belongs to you because it is formed in your opinion. As long as you have that opinion, it will certainly be real. When you no longer believe it, it will no longer be a reality. It is that simple." - Ramtha

"Kindness is a language which the deaf can hear and the blind can read."

Mark Twain

1:14 Goodbye

I, like many others, have always had a problem saying goodbye to people, it seems so permanent. As a youngster I would love visiting people, the word hello meant that the door was open and an adventure was about to start. The next few moments were to be filled with joy and wonder, even it was just catching up with events with an uncle or auntie over a cup of tea. Goodbye meant that the event was finished and the door was closed, it left no room for continuation. Back in my childhood, this formal way of life was the norm in Britain and it was considered rude to behave in any other way. I often would just disappear towards the end of family gatherings rather than say goodbye.

Nowadays we have expressions such as 'see you later' or simply 'later' – both feel more like a comma in a relationship, whereas goodbye is a full stop. I have not used the word goodbye for as long as I can remember. At my son's funeral, during the moments of despair the words 'until we meet again' popped into my mind.

Many years later I was hit like the thunder of one hand clapping by the following text:

> *"Aloha does not mean goodbye. There are no goodbyes in Hawaiian. The concept of separation and endings does not exist in the roots of the original language. In Hawaiian everything is considered alive. The closest thing to goodbye in Hawaiian is ahui ho, which means until we meet again, and more. We will meet again, even if it is in a thousand years, and we will recognize each other's spirit by our eyes."* - William Pila Chiles

'Until we meet again' was the phrase I was searching for as a child, it sums up perfectly my feelings towards a temporary separation. It was served to me by the spirit guardians, a magic elixir that was a hundred times more satisfying than goodbye in my time of need.

Mahalo and blessings

"In matters of style, swim with the current; in matters of principle, stand like a rock."

Thomas Jefferson

1:15 If my body was a car

Scary how true it is!!

If my body were a car, this is the time I would be thinking about trading it in for a newer model.

I've got bumps and dents and scratches in my finish and my paint job is getting a little dull. But that's not the worst of it…

My headlamps are out of focus and it's especially hard to see things up close.

My traction is not as graceful as it once was. I slip and skid and bump into things even in the best weather.

My whitewalls are stained with varicose veins.

It takes me hours to reach maximum speed. My fuel rate burns inefficiently.

But here's the worst of it…

Almost every time I sneeze, cough or splutter, either my radiator leaks or my exhaust backfires!

Source unknown

If my body was a car – what a great analogy! Our body is a highly sophisticated, super computerized vehicle that houses our spirit self, our body of light during our stay here on the physical plane. It is the only one we are going to get in this incarnation, therefore it's very important to look after it. We can, but do we?

A comparison of ways that we look after our car and body is often easier to understand.

New car

People lucky enough to own a new car often start out by returning it to the garage for a regular service, where various basic items are checked and done – replacing oil and air filters comes to mind. The new car is lovingly washed and cleaned every weekend and presented to the world as our pride and joy. We initially pay attention to every detail of that car, but as the novelty wears off, we start to appreciate it a little less, maybe washing it every other weekend, maybe not checking the oil and water so often, and maybe even missing a service to save money. Sooner or later we fall into a poorer routine of care that we feel is the ideal one for our car, we have started to take it for granted. It's at this point that things start to change, and a pattern of care or lack of care starts to emerge and becomes the norm, the accepted substandard level of care. There are five basic levels of standard which we will look at, but first let's go back a step.

The equivalent to a new car is a new body – a baby. Obviously, as a baby we have no control over our bodies or our care, this falls to our parents. Most parents lovingly care and look after their babies – washing, cleaning and feeding their pride and joy. We put new clothes on them, pay detailed attention to their every movement, every smile and every grip; if we have any concerns it's straight down to the doctor. As they start to get older and turn into little children, we also change; maybe we don't pay the same detailed attention, we ask them to clean themselves, and entertain themselves. When they are ill, we might care for them at home and not involve the doctor; this is normal upbringing and it starts to set the standard that the child will adopt when they are old enough to take over the care of their bodies.

There are five basic accepted standards of body care, and all can be related to a car:

1 **Continuum of new car syndrome**
2 **Use it and abuse it**
3 **Use it and fix it**
4 **Wellness**
5 **Professional**

1 Continuum of new car syndrome:

As the title states, this standard is all about a continuation of regular checking of the weekly basics: oil, water, air pressure, cleaning and fueling. Then sending the car in for a service once a year to change oil and air filters. If anything appears to be going wrong, the owner will have it looked at and addressed if necessary.

The average person may not fall into this bracket, mainly because others have been responsible for our care as children, and by the time we take over we have either developed bad habits or want to rebel or experiment. What is the quality of our fuel, our daily food and water, is it healthy or do we fill up on junk food and fizzy drinks? Do we exercise regularly or do we have body weight issues? Maybe we have started to smoke or take drugs, clogging up our air filters and irritating our body systems. Young people who stick to the new car syndrome tend to be gifted sportsmen and women who, due to their sport, check and monitor not only what goes into the body but also how the body reacts to the stresses placed upon it. If anything appears to be going wrong, they will seek professional help as soon as possible.

2 Use it and abuse it:

Unfortunately not only has this become the accepted standard for many people, but it's the fastest growing group. More and more people are spending more and more time in front of TVs and computers, watching and doing unchallenging things. There is an old saying 'Use it or lose it' and when you don't exercise the body and the brain there is only going to be one result. The use and abuse of food, drink and drugs is the curse of western society and often people will take these to the extreme until they destroy the very body that is housing them.

Imagine treating your car this way: driving it badly, over rough ground, hitting things, not cleaning it, not putting in the right fuel, doing no maintenance, running on low tire pressure or worn-out tires. How long do you think the car will keep going before it starts to break down?

Often people get stuck in this syndrome and it takes a wake-up call or a near miss before they take stock and change their lives around. Often the car's engine or body is so bad that it requires professional help to repair and restore it to a level before the owner feels capable of taking control again.

3 Use it and fix it:

This is by far the biggest group. As car owners and drivers, those of us in this group will put in the basics every week and carry out the basic checks; we will even, once in a while, clean the vehicle and keep it tidy. We don't have the car serviced. Instead, the maintenance consists of any issues highlighted at the annual MOT test (compulsory in the UK); tires, brakes and exhaust may have to be renewed to pass this test. In return, we expect the car to start first time every day and get us to our destination and back without breaking down. In short, we have taken the vehicle for granted and have set our standard at a minimum required for essential operation. Most of us in this group are happy with this as an economical exchange. After all, when the car becomes uneconomical we can always buy another one.

For far too many of us this is a normal way of living and treating our bodies. We work hard, eat food that is somewhere between healthy and junk, we have too much coffee, tea and carbonated drinks but also try and have our share of water. We do a moderate amount of exercise, both physical and mental, and probably don't get enough sleep. On top of this we expect our body to keep going day after day; if it breaks down and gets ill we simply see a doctor or take some pills, with the object of getting it up and running again as soon as possible.

4 *Wellness:*

The wellness model is all about taking an enlightened healthy approach to life. It normally comprises people who are middle aged and have taken stock of their lives. This type of person would have deliberately looked for a balanced healthy existence. We try to balance work with rest and play, eat healthily and drink plenty of water without denying ourselves a few treats every now and then. We may undertake a physical and mental exercise routine and visit a bodywork professional on a regular basis. They may be from one of the professions such as a chiropractor, osteopath or physical therapist, or they may be a massage therapist or a complementary therapist practicing their particular brand of therapy. I suspect that most people reading this book will fall into the 'wellness' category.

If we were to relate wellness to a car, these owners would take great care of their vehicle, realizing that the better they look after it, the better it can look after them. They would not only do the basic checks and keep it clean and looking good; servicing and maintenance would be done on a regular basis and at the appropriate mileage rather than towards the end of its life. Items such as tires may be changed before they wear down to the limit as a preventive move. A good care approach is taken throughout the vehicle with an appropriate budget put aside to pay for it.

5 *Professional:*

A professional approach to car care is taken by professional racing teams such as Formula One where after every race every item is removed, serviced, checked and then replaced. Each nut and bolt is undone, lubricated and retightened and set to an exact torque. A computer is placed on each working part to test for maximum performance. The bodywork is cleaned and polished until it is a perfect reflection of the team and sponsor. These cars are set right at the pinnacle of peak performance; however, often the setting is so precise, so near the edge, that one little tweak can cause a breakdown.

In the human body we often see this with professional performers, whether sportsmen and women or dancers. Every element has been covered from nutrition through to exercise and recovery. The body has been built to produce maximum performance in their chosen discipline. Often these people are also supported by a team of professionals, such as nutritionist, fitness coach, doctors, massage therapist and physical therapist. Their training routine will be set to produce the best possible performance at a precise point in time. But as with the cars, it only takes a slight tweak for that to break down, such as a hamstring pull in sprint athletes.

The wellness garage

The wellness garage, if there was such a thing, would be the automobile equivalent of a complementary therapy where a holistic approach would be taken covering mind, body and soul. The Mind, Body & Soul term is normally used very loosely and relates more often as a ripple effect than as a primary interaction. For instance, if we rebalance the wheels of the car, the secondary effect would be to improve the steering by removing the vibration from the steering column and wheel. This in turn will make for a less physically tiring drive for the driver, reducing muscle stress and skeletal compression of the cranium. This removes the likelihood of headaches which improves the health of the driver and ultimately results in a happy owner. So, through the ripple effect, balancing of car wheels can claim to be a holistic approach to car mechanics. A little far-fetched maybe, or is it?

If the garage checked the tires and rebalanced the wheels, re-torqued the steering column, lubricated the steering wheel, massaged the driver and gave them a relaxing half hour in a float chamber, then maybe we have a better claim as a holistic garage because each stage has been turned into primary interaction and the quality of care has improved multifold.

When you drop a pebble into a pond, the immediate explosion of energy produces multiple strong waves all very close to each other; those waves gradually get weaker and slower as they move away from the point of impact. They will gradually slow right down until you can hardly notice them, and then eventually the first weak, energy-less wave will reach the opposite side of the pond. On reaching the other side, thus crossing the whole pond, we can claim to have produced a holistic action: our one pebble has affected the whole pond, at least on some level. On the other hand, if I had five pebbles, and when the power of the first impact started to decrease I threw in another pebble at the point of the decrease, further into the pond, a new more powerful energy would be produced. And if I were to repeat this action as the impact of the second pebble kicked in, an even more powerful energy would emerge, building on the remaining power of the first two. If I was to repeat this right across the pond, imagine the potential for permanent change; this is holistic interaction.

If our mechanics in our wellness garage wanted to produce a service that not only was more productive, more preventive, more holistic, but also one that might bring about a paradigm change to future service of automobiles, it would require more effort, more input, but the effects on the health of the vehicle would be magical.

To produce this new service, our mechanics would look at the technical approach that Formula One teams take with their racing cars. Clearly, it would be uneconomical and not practical to strip down the whole car, but what if we were to undo each nut and bolt a few turns, lubricate it and retighten it to its correct torque? There would be no time lost with misdiagnosis, the introduction of movement and lubrication into the nuts, bolts and their corresponding joints will have a far-reaching positive effect, and the resetting at the correct torque, regardless of whether the presentation was too loose or too tight, would ensure peak performance for that joint within the boundaries of its personal limitations. Each joint would be a new interaction with the car – or a new pebble in the pond – each one building on the increased motion of the other. By this action we could ensure that each car serviced would leave us running and operating as healthily as possible within its own physical boundaries. This is holistic car mechanics.

This analogy is a perfect illustration of how the Starlite® bodycare system works and differs in its technical approach to holistic care. The Starlite® bodycare system is a little bit like an atom – it has a nucleus that is surrounded by a cloud of electrons. The electrons represent all complementary therapies, mixed in a world together but each with its own identity, dancing to its own tune, with its vibration rippling through the rest of the atom. At the core of the Starlite® bodycare system is a nucleus that interacts directly with all of the electrons, a quantum that all complementary healing systems have access to and vice versa. The quantum – 'the minimum amount of any physical interaction of any physical entity involved in an interaction' – aims to systematically dance through the tissues of the body, interacting, lubricating and increasing the range of motion of every joint, ligament and muscle. This results in the maximum potential within the limitations of the individual. When this is coupled with the complementary therapy of choice, the Starlite® bodycare system becomes whole and holistic – a true interaction with universal energy.

*"You must be the change you want
to see in the world."*

MK Gandhi

1:16 The Magic of the Rainbow

Wow!

It's 6.30am on a wet winter's morning and I have just returned from the dreamtime. My first question this morning is "Was that LSD in my curry?" I have spent the night or at least the last few hours dancing and exploring a land of light, in a time of magic. How do I even start to explain who I met?

She/he/it appeared as a mass of color – no, correction, it was interconnecting strands of color, not unlike DNA. A moving, twisting, vibrating essence around a central core of white light, a light so bright that I had to wear three pairs of sunglasses – that's right, three pairs, funny things happen on this side of reality. This 'thing' was not a form that I could recognize or have experienced before, I can only relate to it as 'the essence of color that is the 'magic of the rainbow'.

Communication was through movement of light and a knowing, an instant knowing. We were dancing, there was continuous movement, light and color interacting, expanding and reflecting. We were in a prism, a stargate – the birth place of a rainbow, yet to be dreamed. The prism seemed to be made of a liquid crystal-like substance that appeared to be solid, but wasn't.

'The children of the rainbow want to share these secrets with you. Come, take a look at a small piece of the most wonderful and powerful teaching in the world, a teaching that was once a way of life.'

'Each of us is a spirit in material form. A powerful image for this spiritual truth is the way light interacts with a prism.'

This thought/memory triggered a deluge of information, much of which was lost on the journey home. I looked out from one facet and saw with my mind's eye that:

'The stars are wonderful representations of the light of divine consciousness, the source of light. Starlight is but a twinkle, containing the essence of energy directly from the source of all, a beam of loving and healing white light. Starlight is from the divine source, the source of all energy, therefore by definition is composed of all energy frequencies.'

As the light entered the 'stargate' on its way to the physical world of matter, it met and engaged with 'the essence of color' which before my eyes became a mother, a mother of a newborn rainbow. This beautiful rainbow was different from others – its colors were not separate but entwined. It shone out along a path, a path that contained a lifetime of footprints, my footprints.

As I looked back along the road of the healing arts, I understood – wow! – for the first time I really understood my role, my quest, my destiny.

The rainbow is a bridge that unites, reminding humans how to connect to the realm of light. It represents the path of discovery and enlightenment leading to the other side of the veil (prism) to the pot of gold that contains the beautiful essence of Hawaiian spiritual knowledge.

Science explains that as white light passes through a prism, crystalline structure refracts the exiting light so that it appears as a rainbow spectrum. Each color has a unique frequency and resonates at its own vibration. If the process is reversed, the rainbow once again becomes white light, as each separate part becomes one.

Remember, we are spirit 'sparks of light' – stardancers embodied to have the human experience. The newly embodied stardancers devised a mind and bodycare system that interrogated the healing powers of divine energy. They used pule to open the portal for healing light to travel. They understood the physical division of light and the separation of energy as it passed from spirit to matter.

They then used pule, dance and chants to raise the vibration of each color and weave a beautiful rainbow of healing white light. This was the original lomilomi cosmic system of healing.

The division of color is a representation of modern complementary therapy. The healing arts can be identified as an individual color frequency within the rainbow spectrum. We would find physical therapy and injury rehabilitation at the more solid and slower vibrating end of the rainbow spectrum within the color red. Soft tissue based therapies would be found in orange or yellow. We would find spiritual healing in the higher vibrating opposite end of the spectrum appearing as violet. Psychology would be found in indigo, energy-based therapies in blue and those that claim to work at the interface of energy and structure perhaps in green. All other complementary therapies would be placed somewhere in between. Each holds the essence of the source of healing light.

Without realising it, my path had led me across and around the rainbow, experiencing therapies and learning techniques from every section, every color in the spectrum. Slowly I was weaving my own thread of light around the rainbow. My humble hope is that my single thread can be added to the many others who have responded to the call of aloha and together we can weave a modern rainbow composed of all of the frequencies of light – in balance, in love and in harmony. For surely this must be the way of future medicine.

Huna teaches and science confirms that each color has its own vibration or pattern. In Hawaii colors are always represented as glittering and shining, never still.

Red – commands our every action; it is the color of our physical self, it is used to energize. Care must be taken with this color as it is easy to over energize, causing restlessness. Red boosts our circulation, raises blood pressure and gets our heart pumping faster. If used in an anger situation, it is said that a person is seeing red, or red with rage.

It raises our libido, increases determination, activates our survival instinct and gives us the will to move forward.

Red is the color of physical energy. It is used to energize. Sometimes people have red as a predominant color in their aura. Such people are often warm and affectionate individuals.

Orange – lifts our spirit; freeing our emotions it encourages us to feel liberated and is the color of emotional happiness. Orange gives us the self-confidence and enthusiasm to live our lives with joyful independence. It has a milder effect than red on the circulatory and reproductive systems and is a good color to use for menstrual problems or painful periods as it relieves muscular pain.

This color would be very good for a person who needs more laughter in her life and it is an antidote to depression and loneliness.

Yellow – vibrant rays of sunshine stimulate the intellect; radiating outwards it is the color of the self and the ego. It stimulates our sense of self-worth and empowerment, waking us up to our feelings about others and ourselves. If a person's thinking is confused, yellow would be a good color for them as it helps bring mental clarity and focus.

Pink – combines white (unconditional spiritual love) with red (emotion). Pink would nourish a person who needs a lot of love and nurturing or who has trouble giving love.

Gold – has a quality of performance that no other color has. If someone has a broken bone, lay down lines of gold energy, reconnecting the halves of the break to create a green light for general physical healing. Gold is the color for restructuring. It is also very spiritual; like white light, it represents unconditional spiritual love.

Green – encourages growth, self-love, eases stress and strengthens our inner resolve. It balances, creates harmony and brings us back to our natural center. It bring down blood pressure, calms the heart and nervous system. When concentrations of green are found in an aura, it indicates that healing is taking place there.

Blue – is the color of peace. If someone is disturbed, worried, overexcited, or angry, blue would help to restore calm and peacefulness. It encourages us to communicate our needs, realize our soul's purpose and express our creative self. It is sometimes found as the predominant color of a person's aura, indicating a spiritually inclined, peace-loving individual.

Indigo – is linked to the higher mind and our center of intuition; it gives us the ability to perceive beyond our five senses. It expands our consciousness, encouraging us to peer into unknown realms and gain insights into our everyday lives. Indigo has a calming sedative effect on the body and is a good color to gaze upon before meditation.

Violet – is a mixture of blue and red. In a person's aura it represents spirituality mixed with passion. Sometimes it represents wisdom, which is spiritual knowledge (blue) gained through worldly (red) experience.

Violet inspires our divine will and our spiritual quest in which we desire to experience all that the universe has to offer and to seek answers to philosophical questions. Usually violet is found in significant amounts in a person's aura only when they have reached an advanced level of spiritual growth.

White – has all colors in it, including all the healing colors so it can be used for any kind of healing. It also represents purity, protection, and unconditional spiritual love.

*"We see things not as they are,
but as we are."*

H.M. Tomlinson

1:17 Nail Soup

One day, a man came into a village, and was very hungry. He went to where some women were tending a fire, and said: "Please, ladies, I am hungry and need a pot of water to make some soup."

"But of course, old man, but what are you going to make it with? You don't have any food with you."

The man smiled, and said: "But I do. I have a nail, and it makes the most wonderful soup. I would be happy to share it with you."

The ladies, of course, were sceptical. But soon a pot of water was boiling, and the man pulled out a small, carefully folded piece of cloth.

"Here is the secret to my soup." He opened up the cloth, and pulled out a simple nail. "Now is the time to add it to the water!" With that, he dropped the nail in the pot. "Now my soup is good, but it would be even better if I had an onion or two in it."

"I'll be happy to get you one," said one of the women, "and perhaps I can add a carrot as well?"

"That would be very nice," said the man, and the onions and carrots were added to the pot.

Soon, a small crowd started to assemble. "What are you making?" one of the onlookers asked.

"Why, soup, and it's made with only a nail! It will be delicious."

The onlooker grumbled. "How can soup be delicious when made with only a nail? That's crazy! It needs some beans and potatoes to make it rich. Here, let me get you some." He went away, and returned with beans and potatoes that were quickly added. Seeing this, other villagers came with their gifts of meat, tomatoes and other vegetables. The pot literally overflowed with contributions from the people.

As the pot filled, the crowd grew larger. The soup was ready. Everyone had a bowl and more. As the old man retrieved his nail from the pot, one person in the crowd exclaimed: "Thank you, old man, for your soup. It was the best we have ever had. And to think, it was made with only a nail!" - Scandinavian Folk Tale

"What counts is not necessarily the size of the dog in the fight – it's the size of the fight in the dog."

Dwight D. Eisenhower

1:18 Self-defence

When I arrived she was standing there outside the front of her home with her two-year-old daughter in her arms, with tears running down her face; my young wife had suffered a full day of threatening abuse from a violent and drunken neighbor. Wilber (name has been changed) was celebrating on the day his yearlong restraining order had expired and he was determined to re-establish his perceived power over the neighborhood and in particular those who had stood up to him and said "no more." No more abuse of young children, no more violence to the elderly, no more threatening mind control tactics. Wilber may have just turned 60 years of age, but standing at six foot four and weighing sixteen stone this violent woodsman was still very dangerous, and when goaded on by his two 20-year-old sons he became a raging bull of a man.

Wilber had a long infamous history, tucked away in a wooded corner at the end of the road where he lived with his family, derelict cars and various animals. Over the years he had used baby rabbits to lure schoolchildren into his yard; there he would 'touch' and threaten them, rumors were rife in the neighborhood but the police needed proof in order to take action. Any approach by an angry parent would be met with the threat of violence to their families. Dark winter nights led to bricks going through windows and vehicles being stolen on a regular basis, but no proof could be laid at his doorstep. Then one day while drunk he exposed himself in public to young children while a police officer was visiting a neighbor; he was arrested and charged with a public order offense. After hearing evidence from a small number of brave mothers he received a suspended sentence and was bound over for a year. Now was the time for his revenge, he had found 'the ring leader' and blocked her drive with his truck, he had dumped manure on her car and threatened violence to her children. Her support circle of neighbors had slowly drifted back to the safety of their homes. He became more drunk and aggressive as the day went on. It was the 1980s, there were no cell/mobile phones and no way of contacting me, she just had to be strong and wait for my return.

But what could I do? I was a small slim man weighing only 11 stone, but I loved my family and would walk through fire to protect them. Confronted by the scene of my wife and daughter in danger, I knew intuitively that this was a moment of truth. Face the fear or be controlled by it. Wilber and his two boys were the bullies of the neighborhood and they wanted blood. It was a situation that I had faced many times in the past; when at school I would often jump in to protect a friend and stand up to the bullies, which on most occasions led to a beating and bruising for a few days after. 'Bruised but not beaten' was my schoolboy motto. I had never once turned away from those who would impose violence on the physically weak and I became a thorn in their side, eventually, slowly and reluctantly gaining their respect. In order to reduce the bruising and increase the effectiveness of my protests, I became a student of the martial arts. The most important thing that the training taught me was to keep a presence of mind during a moment of utmost stress; this one tiny piece of wisdom was about to save my life.

Slowly and calmly I approached Sam, the elder of the two boys, and tried to defuse the situation with reasoned argument. But I had made a fatal mistake: by being ignored, the rage of the bull had increased and before I knew what had happened I was suspended in the air, a large hand had me by the throat, its fingers wrapped around my windpipe. At this very moment, time stood still and my mind went into overdrive: red alert!!

During my martial arts training I had developed a color-coded response system; the idea originated from a number of Hollywood films that I had watched. Institutions would be put on 'amber' or 'red alert' – even the Pentagon used a similar warning system. Each warning level has a pre-designed approved level of response; this has many benefits, and first of all, you are not running around like a headless chicken wondering what to do. The approved action has been carefully thought through without any stress element, therefore you can rest assured that the response will be measured and appropriate. You do not have to ask the question, "Is this OK?"

Remember that if you are under attack, you are at a disadvantage. While you are trying to respond with reason to the surprise attack, the attacker has already accepted (in his mind) that it is OK to hurt you. Using a pre-designed warning system allows you to respond without explanation or embarrassment. I had been practicing the alert system for a few years but had never expected to have a red alert.

Red alert, the warning light system of self-defence, had kicked in, there was no time for debate or reasoned response. Red meant action, immediate and decisive action; instinctively I knew I had but one chance and less than a split second to save my life. In slow motion each finger curled in turn creating a fist, a fist that with focused energy became a ball of steel. When Thor's hammer met the jaw of the bull there was only going to be one winner. And then, there was silence. Wilber was swaying six feet away in a mist of bewilderment and confusion, his mind couldn't comprehend what had happened: one minute he was about to swat an irritating fly, the next he was having to deal with the sensation of pain. The two boys, now drugged up on the chemicals of total shock, without a word did exactly what they were told. The truck was removed and the fallen bull taken home to wait for an ambulance. Slowly, neighbors came out of their homes and normality returned to the street. It was a long time before this rage was heard again in the neighborhood and never out in public.

I had learned something new. I grew up believing that violence was not the answer; however, forcible action is a choice and sometimes the only choice. The wisdom was not in the action but in the learning. Whatever you choose to do, do it, believe in it and deliver it with 100% conviction. Anything less would have resulted in failure. Energy and action equals results, and sometimes that action has to be with force.

At first there seems to be a contradiction between being a healer and a warrior; however, many years later I was to learn that they are in fact two sides of the same coin and peaceful warriors do exist.

> *"Both the healing arts and the martial arts of Hawaii were designed to safeguard the O'hana and community."*
>
> Papa Henry Auwae

In ancient times the lomilomi master would also be skilled in lua, a Hawaiian martial art. Their detailed knowledge of anatomy allows them to heal or hurt. They would execute accurate devastating blows, targeting joints and nerves to cause incapacitation. However, their understanding of body language, awareness and attitude allowed them to control a situation without the escalation to physical contact. These skills are needed today as much as they were in the past. We should aim to become a 'Peaceful Warrior'.

It was as a direct result of this incident that the Streetwise self-defence programme for women was launched in association with the local police force. Young mums from many schools were taught street awareness and self-defence techniques; at its core was the 'color alert system of action'.

The color alert system of action. Not every day of your life will be sunshine; somewhere along the road there will be storms of varying magnitude – from light and intense to devastating and life changing. In life we don't go looking for these storms, but being prepared for when they arrive is often the difference between riding the storm or suffering because of it.

We learn CPR and First Aid to be prepared in case we come across a situation where we just might make a difference, even between life and death. Most First Aiders, however, will never use them or may only dip into their skills during their lifetime. The same attitude must be applied to self-defence: if we are to be able to protect our loved ones and ourselves, we must be proficient in the fundamental skill of defence, and defence starts with attitude and awareness.

Awareness:

Awareness is defined as 'having knowledge of something because you have observed it or somebody has told you about it' or 'mindful that something exists because you notice it or realize that it is happening'. In the context of your own personal safety, awareness is the foundation of all your abilities.

Self-defence has three elements: awareness, attitude and combat skills. The first is the most important as 99% of potential situations can be avoided with good awareness.

The Awareness Spectrum:

Your 'life awareness status' can be classified into a spectrum of four colors; each color represents a stage of awareness.

White - Awareness low: rest mode. When in this mode we are normally relaxing at home or in bed. Totally switched off, relaxed, you are looking inward not outward. People in code white when in public are victims in waiting.

Yellow - Awareness switched on: normally. We live most of our life in this mode of awareness. The subconscious is aware of potential danger and will trigger automatic response, with trained muscle memory gained through repetition of movement. When walking down the road you are subconsciously aware of traffic and will avoid being run over. You are calmly and subconsciously looking at your surroundings to assess them for potential threats. You know what and who is around you. Actions such as covering your hand while putting in your pin number, or putting your money away in a bag or pocket before walking out in public. Not leaving your mobile phone on the table of the coffee shop when using the bathroom.

There is a variety of different methods that you can employ to make yourself more aware. Think about assessing everything that comes into a bubble around you. Try imagining you have a radar that pings out and back. Have a commentary constantly running in your head. All these things can help you practice a higher state of awareness. Don't forget this increased awareness needs to be practiced. You can't just change the habits of a lifetime.

Amber - Awareness on high alert. Amber is the state that you go into when something appears not to be right. Your yellow drills have identified something out of the ordinary. Your little voice has started shouting in your ear. Something is wrong; listen carefully because spirit is talking to you. Being on amber alert does not mean that danger is imminent, it simply means that there is a potential for danger and you should draw up plans (in your head) to deal with it. Failing to prepare means preparing to fail.

The most important aspect of the amber code is to set a red line alert. This line can be moved with any changing conditions; it can be reset many times, but never crossed without action. In your mind draw a red line, several shops away from that group of youths who are making you feel uneasy. Then set a plan of action: you may be thinking of exit routes, you may decide to cross the road, you may decide to knock on the door of the house with lights on inside, you may decide to go into a restaurant and call a cab. Decide on your action, and pledge to commit to that action should you reach the red line before the situation changes. If the youths move away or go into a shop, then the situation has changed, the potential danger has been removed for now, and the red line can also be removed, you can continue with your journey. If you feel that the danger has not totally gone – the youths may come out of the shop and start following you – set another red line. You are deciding on the level of threat and danger. Don't ignore the warnings; there is a temptation to 'normalize' these feelings: 'I am just being silly'. Give yourself permission to listen to these feelings, to your gut instinct, to your spirit being; it may just save your life!

Amber prepares you for action, it gives you permission to listen to your feelings and act beyond your level of normality, without embarrassment or apology.

Red - Equals action: it can never be ignored. You are into 'fight or flight' mode and you had better do one or the other quickly. Get up and leave the pub, cross the road, turn around and go the other way, knock on that door and ask for help, call a cab. You have made a choice of action, implement it and stay in charge of the situation. Once action has taken place, a new red line can be set if necessary. Never, ever, forget: if you cross your own red line, you must act positively; failure to do so will impact deeply on your subconscious.

Choice

Many victims of crime or attack have reported that they felt there was something wrong before it happened. All animals, humans included, have highly evolved senses. The problem is that in modern society we often choose to ignore these feelings. We feel stupid or cowardly. We let our egos get in the way. However, this instinct or intuition is there for a reason. It is there to alert us and protect us from danger. An important tool in our awareness bag is giving ourselves permission to listen to these feelings. Don't let ego or conditioning cloud this.

There are many inhibitors to awareness. Alcohol is one of the more obvious. Alcohol clouds judgement and inhibits response. If you are not fit to drive, you are not at your optimum level of awareness. You may be trying to walk home alone. The 'homeward bound' syndrome is another one ruthlessly exploited by rapists and muggers. Women are falling victims to rapists who have found it easier to select a victim from hordes of people carrying bags, briefcases, laptops, or listening to music on their way home from work in the late afternoon or early evening. Your mind is more preoccupied and you are tired. You have slipped into code white.

Awareness is an easy thing in principle, but is more difficult in practice. If you are serious about your personal safety, it is something you must cultivate. Don't become paranoid, just prepared, like installing a smoke detector. Awareness is about seeing, recognizing and identifying risk and threats, and then being prepared to act on them. To maximize your ability to take avoiding action, you must give yourself the best early warning system there is.

Gain Control and Confidence

Control comes from the ability to self-regulate in all circumstances. In a stressful situation people usually either freeze up or overreact. Train and be in touch with your mind and body so that you can deal with all types of conflict in an appropriate and effective manner.

Confidence results from a feeling of certainty. When there is a lack of knowledge or experience about any given subject, then doubt and worry begin to creep into our minds about that subject. Training will help you to understand the processes of conflict which will enable you with a greater sense of self-reliance.

Exercise:

For five minutes stand still with your back to a wall and observe people walking down the street, or in the shopping mall. Look for people who are not taking notice of their surroundings. People plugged into their iPods. People busily texting their friends or chatting on the phone. People happily gazing at the floor, the shop windows or simply contemplating their navels.

These are people with little or no awareness. They are the vulnerable targets and it shows in their body language. If you can spot them, so can others. In its simplest form, this is what you need to avoid. You need to turn yourself into someone not seen as a target. Be confident, be focused and be aware. - Dik Chance

♫ *When the power of love overcomes*
the love of power, ♫
the world will know peace ♫

Jimi Hendrix

1:19 Facing the Bullies (Help for Children)

Once upon a time there was a little boy who was bullied horribly at school. One day it got so bad that he was choked unconscious and the blood vessels in his eyes burst with the pressure. He was the target for constant bullying between the ages of ten and fourteen. Things didn't really change until he grew substantially; the bullies then found an easier target.

His name was David and we had a common bond. Both of us stood out with our blond hair, both of us stood out because we were small, both of us stood out because we had undiagnosed dyslexia, both of us stood out because our families could not afford to buy us long trousers/pants – we attended school in shorts, come rain, wind or snow. This made us different and a target for group bullying.

So when I say I know what you are going through, I really mean it.

"This is remarkably common amongst people who have embraced the reality side of martial arts training. I've met some very, very tough people around the world who were bullied in their youth. That experience seems to have made them stronger and tougher. So, if you are being bullied, take heart." - Dik Chance

Bullying comes in many different forms, and so does defence. I knew someone who became the class clown, thus became popular and no longer a target. He went on to carve out a career in stand-up comedy working the clubs and pubs.

Even though at the time it seems like the end of the world, you will get through it. But you have to start making changes today. How? It's simple: get real, why is someone bullied? Answer: because they are an easy target. What changes do you have to make? Answer: become a hard target. This does not mean become a hard person or even a violent one; it means understanding the bullying situation and then changing it. Remember this: people can only have power over you if you let them.

Institutions such as schools and prisons, sometimes even the workplace, take us back to our lowest common denominator: the fact that we are animals, animals with a pack mentality trying to establish our place in the pecking order. This means that someone will try to have power over you, and you in turn will try to have power over someone else. This is the reality; if you have been bullied, ask yourself have you ever bullied someone, if so why? What did you get out of it? And what made that person your target? This might surprise you and you may have done it without realizing it. But the answers will give you an insight into the mind of a bully and hopefully a course of action.

Unfortunately, you have to take the first steps for yourself. So where do we start?

Understanding why. Most bullies pick on people who are not very confident, showing that they are scared, looking down, talking nervously or too quietly, being timid. Someone who is not going to make a fuss. Someone who appears different because of skin or hair color, wears glasses, fat, thin, tall or small. Has a different level of intelligence. Is rich, poor, or comes from a different social class.

Bullying takes many forms, such as being called names, being ignored and excluded, having things stolen, being pushed, punched, kicked and choked.

Being the target of bullying can leave you feeling confused, helpless, weak and desperate. You can't face leaving the house and may even invent illness to keep you at home. You might feel sick, shaky, weak and in desperate need of the toilet. Your legs might wobble and your hands might be sweaty and shaky. Your mouth might get really dry and all the clever things you hoped to say might get stuck in your throat.

Understanding why. Adrenaline is a hormone that your body produces when you are in an emergency situation. When you are worried at night about something that might happen tomorrow, your body decides this is an emergency and starts to release adrenaline slowly. This makes your heart beat faster and increases your breathing. It can wake you up and can stop you sleeping. When something is threatening you, your body dumps adrenaline into you really fast.

This happens so that your body is prepared for flight (running away) or fight. Unfortunately, if you are not ready for it to happen, it can also make you freeze and panic. Adrenaline is the turbo charge that your body needs in times of danger.

Tell yourself it's just adrenaline and it's your friend.

What can you do? The first thing to do is to accept that it is not your fault. You are not stupid, weak or any other of the negative emotions you are feeling. It is OK to have big ears or glasses or ginger hair or any of the other things that people are using to pick on you. Very often people who are being bullied don't say anything because they are worried what people will think of them. You might even be worrying that you'll make it worse.

Next, start to become a hard target. A hard target is someone who is difficult to get to. The most basic way of being a hard target is to be somewhere else. You can't be picked on if you are not there. If you know where the bullies are going to be, be somewhere else.

We understand what bullies look for when selecting their targets. We can become a hard target by doing the opposite to what they are looking for. What you need to do is show confident and assertive body language, even if you are really afraid inside. We call this duck style. On the surface of the water, a duck looks calm and relaxed. Under the water, its legs are flapping like crazy. It's the same for you. You have to give the impression that you are not nervous and scared, even if under the surface you are flapping like crazy.

So, keep your head and eyes up. You should look confident, strong. Use a strong, confident but polite voice. Walk as though you are going somewhere important.

Do not get involved in conversations with bullies – and remember, keep your distance.

If you have good assertive body language this will go a long way to keeping bullies away. Another trick for your duck style is called 'The Fence'. If you want to keep people out of your garden, you put up a fence. If you want to keep bullies out of your space, you put up your fence. A good fence is just having your hands up in front. It tells the bully you are confident and ready, but it tells people watching that you don't want to fight (so you don't get into trouble too).

Using your confident assertive voice is important too. Don't get involved in bullies' conversations – that's just playing their game.

Just put up your fence and say: "What do you want?" over and over, just like a stuck CD. If you are not responding, their game plan isn't working. If that isn't working and they are getting too close to your 'fence' tell them to BACK OFF loudly. - Dik Chance

All of this makes you a hard target, and all things being equal the bully will look for an easier target.

If you are a target, you will need to move to the next level of understanding a bully and think smart. Bullies talk in a language that consists of two elements: a demand and a threat. Do this and that, don't do this and that, give me this and that, or I will... They are gambling that the threat to you is greater than their request from you.

Their language also identifies their weakness; ask yourself why that object or action is important to them. If you are of a different race or culture, are they afraid of the unknown? If you are seen as weak, stupid, ugly, or any other negative things, are they afraid of being associated with that same quality and therefore losing face within their peer group? 'Don't tell the teachers, the police, and your parents' – all of these statements mean that the bully is afraid of being found out. Do you see a pattern emerging? Ultimately the bully is afraid that you will in some way expose his/her weakness – remember, all bullies are cowards!

Every bully at some stage will have told you not to tell the authorities – why? Answer: because they are afraid. Therefore the first thing you should do is tell someone.

It is vital that you tell someone. To start with, you might feel comfortable telling your friend. That's OK. You might feel a little safer if you are not on your own. However, if the bullying is continuing, you need to tell someone who can do something about it. Speak to your parents, another family member, a friend or a sympathetic teacher.

Keep a record of everything done or said to you. Childline has an excellent log that you can download.

By telling an adult, you have asked them to help you with the problem. Adults should listen to you and they have ways of helping available to them that you may not have. Schools should have anti-bullying policies that they should use to help stop the problem. If the problem doesn't stop, tell someone else. Speak out and speak out loudly. Don't forget that bullies look for someone who is not going to make a fuss. Tell someone, make a fuss and you become a hard target.

Huna

The way of aloha…

The world is what you think it is.

There are no limits.

Energy flows where attention goes.

Now is the moment of power.

Love is to be happy with.

All power comes from within.

Effectiveness is the measure of truth.

1:20 Simply Huna

Huna is based on the seven principles listed above; it is the science of making things happen. You can live a rewarding and fulfilling life simply using Huna as a guide.

It is not my intention in this book to explore the depths of Huna — that requires its own book and there are already many excellent ones out there. I am simply bringing it to your attention as the philosophy plays an integral part in lomilomi massage and bodycare.

I would implore you to read a book or two on the subject in order to get an understanding, then seek out a world-class teacher. For those who are just starting to explore the teaching of Huna there are a number of good books in the bibliography section at the back of this book; I have met many of the authors and can recommend their works. On this page I am going to refer to one such person who has an extraordinary knowledge on the subject. Over the years I have been fortunate enough to have attended several seminars by Serge Kahili King held in Europe and the US.

To get you started, here is a sequence of sayings designed by Serge Kahili King which can be used every day to remind you of the philosophy, to clear the mind, to stabilize and harmonize emotions, and clarify purpose ready for the day's activities. The important thing is to take a moment before your day begins to ready yourself for the successful day you will be creating.

Be aware~ that the world is what you think it is. Decide that you have the power to succeed.

Be free~ because there are no limits. Give yourself the right to succeed.

Be focused~ because energy flows where attention goes. Increase your desire to succeed.

Be here~ because now is the moment of power. Start right now with a will to succeed.

Be happy~ because love is the source of power. Enjoy and acknowledge the good that is.

Be confident~ because all power comes from within. Always trust yourself.

Be positive~ because effectiveness is the measure of success. Always expect the best.

"Everything is told, no secrets are kept."

Serge Kahili King

The way of aloha

Huna is a modern name for an ancient system of esoteric knowledge and practice. It is a system that uses the power of the mind in order to influence nature and events. It has been referred to by many names, such as: the way of the sacred light; the secret; the knowledge of the inner world. Today it's simply Huna.

The seven principles are just like gravity, in use every day and works whether you believe in it or not. So why not gain an understanding, apply the knowledge and take control of your life? Huna has many levels, many layers and can be as simple or as deep as you want it to be.

My understanding of Huna is a very simple one and I try to apply it every day; the results have been nothing short of astonishing.

This is my simple understanding of how things unfold on a daily basis.

You don't wake up in the morning, lie in bed and decide whether you are going to be in a good mood or a bad mood, whether it's going to be a good day or a bad day. What normally happens to the majority of us is that we allow ourselves to be influenced by some external stimulus. That stimulus can be positive on a global or local level, such as the opening of the Olympic Games or waking up to a bright sunny day – this tends to put us in a good mood and the day unfolds in a positive way. Conversely, if the stimulus is negative on a global or local level, such as the recession is getting worse, more jobs are being lost or waking up after a bad night's sleep, this will tend to put you in a bad mood and the day unfolds in a negative way.

Why?

Because the external stimulus is picked up by our sensory system, we hear it and we see it. That produces a thought in our mind; the thought starts a chemical reaction in the pituitary gland at the base of our brain. The chemical or hormone allows us to experience the thought in physical terms. If it's a bad or unhappy thought, we will feel sad, maybe depressed, we may produce tears of sadness, our musculoskeletal body will respond by maybe dropping the head forward, rolling the shoulders forward, we may hold our head in our hands, we may walk in a slow heavy manner. We may shut the world out, close down and go into a protective mode. The physical manifestation of the negative makes us feel bad, and when we feel bad we tend to notice other negative things in order to enhance this experience. That in turn produces a thought which starts a chemical reaction... I think you know what comes next, this is a vicious circle.

The same process happens to a positive or happy thought which starts a chemical reaction in the pituitary gland at the base of our brain. The chemical or hormone allows us to experience the thought in physical terms. This time we have a smile on our face, we feel uplifted, we walk with a spring in our step and joy in our hearts, we stand tall and hold our head up, we open up to the world and to those around us, and the world looks and feels great. We tend to notice little things such as children or dogs playing, music coming from a bar, or simply the sun shining and the birds singing – all of these things will enhance the experience of feeling good. 'Today is a good day' – wait a minute, is that not a thought on its way to the pituitary gland?

The mind does not class a thought as good or bad; it's just a thought and is embraced as part of the great human experience. Like attracts like; if you are in a low (sad) dense vibration, you will tend to attract more of the same in order to enhance the experience. The same applies to a high (happy) light vibration, it's just energy.

Now I will let you into a secret: it is impossible to be happy and sad at the same time. Do you get that? It is impossible to be happy and sad at the same time.

Therefore why not take control of your life and decide how you want to spend your day?

I start my day with a simple morning affirmation (wilful, conscious intent) which lifts and sets my mood, my outlook and inevitability my day. And the fantastic thing is that when in the right mindset you can ride even the hardest knock.

I also start my sleep with a simple evening reflection of gratitude (for the day's lessons, gifts and blessings). The funny thing is I now tend to rise in the mornings with a bright outlook, no matter what the weather or day's schedule might hold.

If you are a glass half empty person, flick the switch and start thinking in terms of half full. Stop moaning about things you don't have and start appreciating the things you do have, for every one of us has won more lotteries than we can possibly imagine. We are all winners – start behaving like one and live life to the full.

Simple Huna:

The world is what you think it is~ wake up in the morning and decide how you want your day to be, you choose.

Energy flows where attention goes~ remember, like attracts like. You choose what you want and focus on it.

There are no limits~ you can be as happy or as sad as you want to be, it's your choice.

Love is to be happy with~ aloha is love and acceptance, implement the principles above, live the way of aloha, and happiness and contentment is assured.

All power comes from within~ it all starts with a thought, you decide which one.

Now is the moment of power~ start now... right now!

Effectiveness is the measure of truth~ use this formula every day for a month, it has the power to change your life.
I guarantee that you will never be the same again.

1:21 Rules for being Human:

1 *You will receive a body* – you may like or hate it, but it will be yours for the entire period of this time around.

2 *You will learn lessons* – you are enrolled in a full-time informal school called life. Each day in this school you will have the opportunity to learn lessons. You may like the lessons or think them irrelevant and stupid.

3 *There are no mistakes, only lessons* – growth is a process of trial and error. Experimentation. The 'failed' experiments are as much a part of the process as the experiment that ultimately 'works'.

4 *A lesson is repeated until learned* – a lesson will be presented to you in various forms until you have learned it. When you have learned it, you can then go on to the next lesson.

5 *Learning lessons does not end* – there is no part of life that does not contain its lessons. If you are alive, there are lessons to be learned.

6 *There is no better than here* – when your 'there' has become a 'here', you will simply obtain another 'there' that will again look better than 'here'.

7 *Others are merely mirrors of you* – you cannot love or hate something about another person unless it reflects something you love or hate about yourself.

8 *What you make of your life is up to you* – you have all the tools and resources you need. What you do with them is up to you. The choice is yours.

9 *Your answers lie inside you* – the answers to life's questions lie inside you. All you need to do is look, listen and trust.

10 *You will forget all this.*

Cherie Carter-Scott

"Whether you think you can or think you can't, you're right."

Henry Ford

1:22 Words have Power

One day at our busy birth trauma clinic, I was introduced by a midwife from King's College Hospital in London to a young mum who had been diagnosed with Bell's palsy (facial paralysis resulting from a dysfunction of the cranial nerve VII).

Apparently, the patient was undergoing a Cesarean operation in order to remove the baby from the womb when she became conscious and the shock of the event resulted in facial paralysis. It was one of the worst cases I had seen, with a severe contusion of the facial muscles, the closure of one eye, the drying of the tear ducts, a constant dribbling of saliva and a continuous mild pressure headache.

On top of this, the patient was unable to look at herself in the mirror or show her face to any child as their reaction confirmed her belief of feeling ugly. This led to depression and hopelessness, which in turn triggers the pituitary gland to produce hormonal chemicals reinforcing the negative feelings; she was trapped in a continuous downward spiral.

The consultant had told her that most Bell's palsy conditions should start to improve in 12 months or so, and she should concentrate on looking after the baby and not be so self-conscious. Clearly, he was not going to offer any further help. What's more, his negative comments appeared to have made the condition slightly worse due to the rise in anxiety. Recently the term placebo was inverted into a new term, nocebo, to describe the negative effects of a doctor's opinion. We know from placebo that if the patient has an acceptance of possibility – act well and be well – the chemical balance will follow (Dopamine/Parkinson's experiment). Conversely, negative comments and thoughts lead to the corresponding chemicals being released.

The young lady (who we shall call Emma) originated from Columbia, worked as an office cleaner and could not afford chiropractic treatment. However, after a personal request from the midwife, who was a regular client at our clinic, I agreed to meet and help as part of a research project into the mind-body link. Clearly, the trauma had been triggered by the mind and therefore I reasoned that maybe the solution to healing would be also found in the same area.

On the anatomical side of the equation, it is thought that an inflammatory condition leads to swelling of the facial nerve. The nerve travels through the skull in a narrow bone canal beneath the ear. Nerve swelling and compression in the narrow bone canal are thought to lead to nerve inhibition, damage or sometimes even death.

Physical therapy can help to maintain muscle tone and stimulate the facial nerve. It is also important that muscle re-education exercises are introduced along with soft tissue mobilization techniques to prevent permanent contractures of the paralyzed facial muscles.

Now the real turning point for Emma came six weeks after the birth of her child, when Linda, her caring midwife, convinced her that we had the skills and could help her overcome the horrendous position she found herself in. Her arrival at our clinic signified that a) she wanted and was ready to engage into the healing process, and b) she believed that we could help her achieve this.

As stated, the physical therapy side of the equation was very important – first for the physical reasons mentioned above, but equally important for the placebo effect, her belief that we were 'doing something' that would eventually result in the return of her facial features and the control of those features. This triggered the very chemicals required to start the healing process. Remember, emotion follows thought, and emotion triggers a chemical release from the pituitary gland to reflect the original thought. At the very least, our positive actions would combat her original negative view.

My approach, beliefs and experience were now going to be tested in full view of Emma's family, Linda and the midwives from King's, and their consultants. You see, for many years the medical profession, and indeed many of my colleagues, dismissed placebo as being 'all in the mind'. My argument to them was simple: if it's all in the mind and it works, then the power of the mind must be enormous and surely we are missing a trick by dismissing it. Placebo could be the key to finding the healing 'magic' that we are all looking for.

I love the word magic; it implies something mysterious, something wondrous, some elusive power beyond the limits of the world. Magic in reality is tomorrow's science not yet understood.

Emma would only leave her house covered head to toe; she would get into her husband's car and did not show her face in public. I told her that she could come to my private studio at my home for treatment.

As stated, the real healing started with a change of belief from hopelessness to hopefulness. I started by taking a full medical record from Emma. We spent over an hour, one-to-one, doing this. We explored her fears and her passions; I had empathy but not sympathy, she was already drowning in that, but the real benefit could be found in the development of the rapport between us.

I took a calm rational approach, explained the physics behind our techniques and portrayed an air of total confidence in the outcome (remember the duck syndrome). This alone produced positive changes: within two days the headache had stopped, and the facial contusion was softer.

Over the next few weeks, three in total, during our sessions I re-introduced Emma to herself – not her physical self but to her loving spirit. She fell for my dog Max who licked her face with unconditional love; we chatted and laughed about her daughter, and I constantly told her that her facial expression was improving and that her physical beauty was returning. Everything we did (and by we I mean my family, including the dog) was to induce feelings of love, laughter, happiness and worthiness in Emma; after all, 'energy flows where attention goes'. I wanted her to be fully committed to healing herself, consciously and subconsciously, fully committed, mind, body and soul, to producing positive chemical hormones. If I was the conductor, then Emma was the orchestra and the energy of grace was the sweet music producing the healing that we were experiencing.

Three weeks after our first meeting, Emma looked into a mirror and smiled a half smile; if there is magic then we had been dancing to its tune. Once again, Emma's eyes sparkled as tears appeared – this time, though, they were tears of happiness. To me they were worth much more than any monetary return, they were a treasure that would bring a lifetime of smiles.

It was to be another two weeks before Emma had 99% of her functions back. Placebo, the power of love, the power of belief – you choose. Emma and I know that there is magic beyond the limitations of science.

The view of Emma's consultant was that it would have happened anyway!

The only thing stopping the exploration of the unlimited mind is the limited mind of the explorers.

"I am everything, created and uncreated I am the Universe..."

Aham Brahmasmi

1:23 Transformation

We are spirit bodies here to have the human experience – the earth is not our home, it's our classroom, a divine school of esoteric studies, the university of life, for gaining experience, knowledge and growth.

In order for that experience to be authentic, we pass through a veil that wipes clean our soul memory for the duration of our visit. We temporarily forget our true nature, that we are reflections of light, spirits of divinity transported from the dreamtime into this physical existence. During each lifetime, our immortal soul through embodiment has an opportunity for spiritual growth and to expand its level of consciousness before returning to join and enhance the matrix of creation.

The Law of Conservation of Energy states: 'Energy (or its equivalent in mass) can neither be created nor destroyed'. Given that we are energy beings who exist in the universe, we must all abide by this law. A denial of our energy privileges affects us on all levels of existence – physically, emotionally, mentally, spiritually, and mystically.

> *"To avoid criticism do nothing,*
> *say nothing, be nothing."*
>
> Elbert Hubbard

1:24 The Ugly Duckling
A world of gray

One of my very first memories as a baby was one of a gray world, a world without color. My first intellectual memory was that of a baby in arms, no more than six months old. I can recall the scene: it must have been winter, the sky was gray, even the air around me seemed to have a gray consistency to it, there were people everywhere, on the pavements and standing at bus queues, they were gray people, they had pale complexions

and were dressed in gray. Just like an old black and white film, there was no color!

I remember clearly taking in the whole scene before me and thinking to my baby self: this is OK, now all I have to do is to keep the knowledge of who I am and where I came from. This thought came from a baby who relied on his mother to pick him up, to feed him, to clean him, and to love him; the only way he could communicate was with his eyes, the mirror to his soul.

Inevitably, as the baby me concentrated on survival in the world of flesh and bone, learning to communicate with sound and movement, and trying to get to grips with his new embodiment, I soon forgot who I was, where I had come from, and even why I was here.

However, that first scene of a gray world remained forever etched on the memory, to be visited again later in life. That one memory confirmed many things:

◆ *That I and others have intelligent thought as babies.*

◆ *That we have a clear knowing.*

◆ *Making a choice to come here for a purpose.*

◆ *The existence of another place, another dimension, home, the place where we lived when we made the choice to come here.*

◆ *Previous life experience: if I thought that 'this incarnation was OK' then I must have had some knowledge or experience to compare it with, something that was not OK.*

I recently shared this memory with my 80 year-old mother, who added her story to the scene. She was in her early twenties when I was born. My parents rented rooms in an old Victorian building in South London. It was just over ten years after the Second World War had finished, there were bomb sites everywhere and food rationing had only just stopped. On weekdays my mum would take me from our apartment in a tenement block on the short walk to the subway station; there we would catch a train to my grandma's house, where my mother would leave me while she went to work in the city. At the end of the day, we would make the same journey in reverse.

The winter months in post-war London were hard living. There was no heating, only coal fires which resulted in a fog of heavy pollution; sometimes it was so thick that you could only see an arm's length in front as you walked through the early evening darkness. Everyone wore long dark gray overcoats and hats. Any light, natural or artificial, was diffused by the fog; indeed it was a gray world and as far as color was concerned, it truly was the ugly duckling part of my life.

The sun brings with it warmth, light and color to the world – oh to live in a land of eternal spring! But then again, without experiencing the dark winter months how can we truly appreciate the bright summer months? Throughout my life I would seek the sun; many of us who live in the high northern hemisphere are affected by SAD (Seasonally Affected Disorder) and as you get older, attraction to the sun gets stronger as you constantly turn from the dark gray to the world of eternal color.

The world of color

All children love rainbows and painting with colors. I was no exception; painting with color in our primary school was a joy, but I don't remember color coming into my physical world until I was 12 years old and we moved to the suburbs where I was to experience green trees and fields, yellow daffodils – even the sky changed from white/gray to blue.

But of course I had access to color every day in the dreamtime, a world vibrant with energy, color and life. A place where I would meet my animal friends and explore the virtues of color and the vibration of energy they produce. Just like any other message received by the senses, color affects emotion, emotion triggers chemicals, and chemicals affect the body.

> *If you talk to the animals, they will talk with you and you will know each other.*
>
> *If you do not talk to the animals, you will not know them, and what you do not know you will fear.*
>
> *What one fears, one destroys...*
>
> Chief Dan George

1:25 Power Animals

I have and have had a group of power animals or animal helpers with me all my life; they often appear at times of need. Until I started to study shamanism I simply accepted these as imaginary friends that all children have, mine just happened to stay with me into adulthood. Different animals have come to me at different times of my life or on different occasions, but always the right one for the occasion would appear. I have never been let down by an animal helper or spirit, here is a story about some of those spirits.

My parents had four children and I was the eldest. From an early age I was given the responsibility of looking after my brother and sisters; as a result, taking responsibility and leading others became quite natural for me. These assets were recognized when at the age of 12 I joined the Boy Scouts where I was quickly promoted to become what was at the time the youngest patrol leader in the county. It was in the Scouts that my power animal allies really came alive, especially at camps and adventure treks. These were great carefree times for any young kid to have experienced. Our inner city upbringing was in complete contrast to the adventures in the Scouts: we would spend our days in the woods, or canoeing down a Welsh river then set up camp on the river bank. The evenings would be spent singing Kumbaya around the camp fire while eating hot sausages – happy days.

One Easter our whole Scout troop was trekking through the Brecon Beacons in Wales. We had set up camp as usual, only this day was different: our leaders had decided that a patrol made up of senior Scouts (I was the youngest) would do a night mountain trek. It was a lovely warm evening and the moon was shining as we left but after a couple of hours the climb started to get steeper and the clouds thicker, reducing the moonlight to shadows. One of our number called Barrie lost his footing and twisted his ankle; we improvised by supporting him and carried on at a slower pace. Before long it became obvious that moving at the slower pace we would not reach our destination and support vehicles on time. A decision was made to leave a small group behind with the injured Scout with the rest proceeding on to the rendezvous to get help (there were no mobile/cell phones in the 1960s). I was left in charge of the small group with the injured Barrie and we set about finding some shelter by the side of the track; this shelter was little more than a thicket. The clouds were getting thicker, and the moonlight was fading; just then the heavens opened up and none of us had any waterproof equipment.

The rain got heavier and the night darker, it wasn't long before we were soaked through and one or two started to shiver. My orders were to stay and wait for help; this we did, however, the situation had now changed and we were in danger of getting hypothermia before any help arrived. I reassessed the situation: we were possibly a little over halfway to the rendezvous, and we had no way of knowing if the other group were going to meet the support vehicles before they left, let alone get help back up the mountain on time. I calculated that if we waited 20 minutes more we would be at the point of no return, the point where we would not have control over our destiny. We were exposed to the elements and hypothermia was now a very real possibility. I decided that we needed to move, movement would create energy which in turn would become body heat, and it would also raise our spirits. But which direction should we go in? Both were gambles. Forward, and if we were lucky we might meet a rescuing party if the other group did manage to get through on time, if not there would be no one to meet us. This would be the only direction that any help would come from. However, we also did not know what surprises the route had in store: ditches and new streams due to the heavy rainfall – and there was now no moonlight, only a short beam from our one fading flashlight. If we turned back the way we came, we would at least know the route, maybe recognize landmarks, thus have an idea of distance and we could guarantee that there would be people at base camp if we got there. On the down side we would be walking away from any possible rescue.

As we took the first positive step towards our survival, the words popped into my head: 'I am the captain of my ship, I am the master of my fate'. Where they came from I don't know, but there he was, the essence of a wise owl, I could feel him in my head right behind my eyes, I could see with his eyes piercing through the wind and rain, then he whispered: "When you let the light in, you can see in the dark." It would be so easy to wander off the path in the darkness and end up in some crevasse, but the spirit of the owl stayed with me, lighting up the path. It was as though I had infra-red night vision; step by step I led our small group down the mountain track back towards the rest of our lives.

When recalling this story for the book, I realized that by coincidence the name of that patrol was 'the owls' – but then again, there are no coincidences!

Owl – In years to come the eyes and wisdom of the owl would be there for me on many occasions. Sometimes during my chiropractic studies I would have to attend a student clinic in Cardiff. This would entail getting up at 2am, driving the 176 miles to Cardiff in Wales and being ready for a 9 o'clock public clinic. We would have a full day, finishing our clinic duties at 6pm; we would be cleaning up and leaving at 7pm for a long drive home. This could be particularly stressful during the dark winter months. I would always take a few minutes out before driving home, have a quick wash and freshen up, then ask my owl spirit to sit with me and guide me on the way home. His eyes were all seeing, his concentration was always sharp, I felt like I was a fighter pilot on maneuvers flying with clear night vision, I missed nothing, every detail was noticed, it was as though my concentration and ability were operating at another, far superior level. On my arrival home, I always thanked the owl for his presence and for traveling with me.

Dreamtime: *The owl is the doorway into the unknown; she lives between the worlds and can bring light into dark places. Night is a time of rest for most creatures, but in the presence of the moon, when the trees are sleeping and everything is in repose, you can change things. You can recast the pieces of your life, feel where shifts occur and become aware of all aspects of the power of change.*

Tiger – I have two power animal tiger spirits, both completely different.

The first one is a small young cub called Kiki, he is always bouncing around full of fun, youth and life. This essence often visited and played with me from about the age of two, his strongest presence was during my teen years, but he still comes back and joins in the fun, especially when the family, my granddaughters or children are around. He almost feels like the spirit of my eternal youth; when he comes to play I can put all the pressures of life and the responsibilities of being an adult to one side for a while and become a child again.

The other essence is courageous, strong and fearless. This tiger helper is an adult she or he – the spirit is a combination of male and female and appears in time of danger. She is definitely a protector, a guardian, and has got my blind side covered and I absolutely trust it with my life.

This tiger spirit came to my rescue one day over 20 years ago when I was up the top of a ladder trying to clear our gutters and downpipes which had become clogged up with autumn leaves causing the rain to flow over the top. I happened to overreach, causing the ladder to slide on the plastic gutter. It moved about one foot and stopped only because of a joint bracket, and the fact that I had managed to grab hold of the gutter with my left hand and onto the ladder with my feet meant that I was anchored one way while the ladder was caught in the other direction. All this was being played out nearly 40 feet up from the ground. At times like these your mind goes into hypersonic speed, assessing the situation and trying to decide between fight, flight or freeze. A wave of fear comes over you that is so strong – often worse than the situation you are in – that you will do almost anything for that feeling to go. I clearly remember my brain telling me that it needed to get rid of the fear fast and this could be achieved by just letting go (flight) and not prolonging the agony. A split second later, the tiger spirit appeared in my mind. She was cool and calm and with complete authority she told me to "take a deep breath, relax, it's going to be all right, take another deep breath and using all your strength pull yourself and the ladder back to the center of the gutter." All of a sudden I had no fear, I took the deep breath and pulled myself back. Slowly, step by step, I came down from the ladder, thanked my guardian angel – the tiger spirit – let her go and then began shaking with the realization of the situation.

Dove – she is known to me as Little Dove and is with me during times of great sorrow.

He was only three days old when he died, does that make the pain any less? Only those who have lost a child are qualified to answer.

It was midnight when the phone rang; I was tired and slept through it. Next there was a knocking at the door; when I looked out of the bedroom window I could see the blue lights and uniformed police officers. Only two weeks before, my wife was celebrating her 20th birthday, now she was being rushed into the operating theater for an emergency Cesarean section to try and save her life and the life of our baby son. Premature and weighing just 3lb. he simply was not strong enough to survive. He lived for three days but remains forever in our hearts. My wife Sandra had to stay in hospital for observation for a week or so; I had to go through the painful process of registering a birth with the authorities while at the same time arranging a funeral. I spent the days visiting Sandra and organizing; however, in the evenings and early mornings I had to deal with the fact that the first ever funeral that I was going to attend was that of my own son.

It was during this period that Little Dove appeared as wispy white light in the shape of a bird. She would fly into my dreamtime, she would then sit with me radiating love and smiling with a knowing look in her eye, it was as though she understood what I was going through. When she was there I felt comforted, I felt as though I was being cradled by the hand of divine love. And those eyes, they reminded me of...

...an imaginary childhood friend, someone who has been with me throughout my life, caring, nurturing, loving, could it be...

Nowadays Little Dove travels in and out of my life on the tip of the wind, and she comes in the form of white light in a bird shape, but transforms into a beautiful Indian lady.

She is the lady of mercy who can touch your heart, through love and tender care. She is a lady who has seen pain and misery, far beyond her teenage years. I feel a deep connection with her, perhaps I know her from a previous life, or perhaps I know her simply because she wants me to know her. She has told me that she knows my pain because we have shared pain. She can love because we have shared love. She can forgive as I must learn to forgive. She can show mercy because she has experienced the extremes of no mercy; I know that her brief existence in human form had ended in butchery, an act so violent and her forgiveness so sincere that love was transfixed in time and her spirit transformed into the wings of mercy.

If ever I find it hard to forgive those who have done me wrong, I ask Little Dove for help and advice. She has a way of showing me another way to view a situation or person. And whenever I have a great time, a happy day or a deep loving emotion, I share the experience and loving energy with her.

Bear – For me the bear has been a giver of strength and protector of space. Have you ever felt overwhelmed with the number of people around? Have you ever been pushed and shoved in a large crowd? It's at times like these that I ask my bear spirit for help. With the bear I simply close my eyes, breathe in deeply a few times and welcome into my body the spirit of the bear. The bear appears to me clearly as a vision of a big brown bear; I can not only see him, but I can also touch and feel him, he has a sense of curiosity around me. On his arrival I can physically feel my body change; I am only a small person, but with the bear spirit in me I feel six feet tall, big, heavy and muscular. Now a funny thing happens with the help of the bear: the bear will occasionally let me breathe in his essence, I can then slowly and purposefully walk through a crowd and the crowd all separate to let me through, there is no pushing or shoving. I have experimented with this on many occasions – it always works. Some days I have to travel into the center of London during the rush hour, my train will arrive at platform 15-17 which is in the far corner of Victoria station, the underground is on the opposite side of the concourse. This inevitably means walking diagonally across the crowd with all the resulting bumps and excuse me's. Most days I simply accept the hustle and bustle of life. Sometimes, however, if I feel a little closed in, I might ask the bear for help ten minutes before we arrive at the station and on those occasions I never have problems from the crowd.

Chameleon – When attending workshops I adopted a persona that would blend into the background. I didn't want special treatment, positive or negative, from the tutor; I wanted to be seen and treated as just another student. To achieve this I had to avoid extremes that would make me stand out – extremes of opinion, of experience, of education, of knowledge. I found that the best way of blending into the background was with the help of my friend the chameleon. When I first came across the problem of how to present myself at workshops in order to obtain the purity of the teaching, I asked the universe for help. This resulted in an introduction to my friend the chameleon during a shamanic dream, who presented me with a long coat of many colors. When I am wearing this coat I can adapt to any situation and blend into the background; it helps to suppress the ego and any self-promotion while at the same time letting in all relevant information. Before each workshop I simply ask my friend the chameleon to let me borrow his coat, and with this coat my mindset is that of just another student. After each workshop I clean the coat, removing any old energy, and return it to the chameleon with thanks and blessings.

Dolphin – Azura, the lady of twilight has appeared, she is a mixture of shimmering white/silver light with hues of ocean blue radiating from a smoke-like form somewhere between a mermaid and a dolphin. She travels between the worlds of spirit and matter. Her first words to me were "I share the wisdom of all that is, learn true communication and share this wisdom with others."

To me she is the keeper of sacred knowledge; it is the knowledge of the ocean, traveling on cosmic waves through a sea of possibilities in the infinite ocean of potentiality. She understands the rhythm of life and the power of breath to release emotions. She represents change and wisdom, balance, harmony and freedom.

Ancestral knowledge passed down from Hawaiian elder Hale Makua states that dolphins are the embodiment of the high guardians that accompanied our light souls during the migration across the cosmos 18.5 million years ago. They stayed as embodied beings so that they would be here when we were ready to receive the knowledge of our purpose and our destiny.

> **Dreamtime:** *Dolphins are extremely sensitive, playful, uninhibited spirits who can teach us a lot about the pure joy of life. They are intelligent caring beings who can communicate telepathically with those who are tuned in. Dolphins perceive reality as one thing melding into another; they are absolutely present within each moment. By swimming in the dolphin's world, appreciating simplicity and feeling the joy of leaping out of water into the completely alien world of air, we receive a model, a way of experiencing our lives that gives a strong assurance of the ultimate continuance of everything that occurs.* -
> **Dreamtime from Power Animal Meditations by Nicki Scully**

Wolf – A lone gray wolf wandered into my spirit world just as I was questioning my future direction. I was coming to the end of my bodywork jigsaw quest, what was I supposed to do now? Do I share it or use it and if so how? I had been in private practice and a practical tutor at the chiropractic college and postgrad mentor; I have run workshops, trained football teams and run a karate club. Now, though, I doubted my ability to communicate and teach on an intellectual level; some days dyslexia can make you tongue-tied, word blindness can hit you at any time. I wasn't sure if I was the best person for this.

"Who are you?" I asked.

"It is simple who I am. I am the voice. You see, there are many components in the spirit realm. The voice is the teacher. It is what you are – a wolf.

It is what they seek, the one who knows, the voice, the path. Some refer to it as education. Some refer to it as intelligence. Some refer to it as knowing. Some refer to it as the great understanding, the spiritual path and the voice opens the way.

You are a wolf, and a wolf has a complex method of communicating which involves body language and vocal skills. If you have a problem expressing your thoughts, needs or ideas to others, take time to study another wolf. For the medicine of a wolf will help you gain your objectives through cooperative endeavors. I have entered your life because it is time for you to share knowledge and information. You have the authenticity and the power to teach." - Wolf Moondance

Dreamtime: *Wolf helps you see the truth of where you are at the moment and gives you guidance that is pertinent to where you are headed. You can trust that it is always safe to work with him. You can always count on him to give you authentic reflection of yourself.*

If I ever doubt or need reminding of my purpose, I simply put my hand in my pocket and pull out a card with the following words on it:

Discovering your mission puts you in a position of responsibility.

From this point on you must act as a torchbearer for others who still struggle with their spiritual identity.

Your life must be a testament that anyone can do as you have done.

Attracting Power Animals – The stories above are just some of the power animals that I have had the pleasure to share my present incarnation with. You will find that the more you communicate with these animal spirits, the more that they and others will be attracted to you. One of the best ways to attract power animals is to have a good relationship with animals in the physical world. If you find that animals are naturally attracted to you, it may be because they recognize the presence of your spiritual energy.

Animals are more sensitive to energy than people and instinctively recognize a kindred spirit, and if you are into complementary therapy and the healing arts, try learning animal communication, the trust technique, animal Reiki or Laulima. Animals understand the healing potential contained within energy techniques that will help to maintain their health on a mental, physical and emotional level, allowing them to be happy, peaceful, relaxed, healthy, calm and stress-free.

We have always had dogs at home ever since I can remember. I have lived and played with these beautiful, energetic and loving creatures, I seem to have a natural affinity with them. My mum recently told me that when I was a youngster I often said it's because I was a dog before I came here. On a number of occasions I have been warned to be careful by the owner of an apparently aggressive dog, a dog that does not like men. Then, much to the owner's surprise, a few minutes later the dog and I are playing like long lost buddies.

You will find that as your skills develop, your relationships in the physical world with animals will deepen. As a direct result, you will attract more power animals from the spirit dimension; this is a natural occurrence, just concentrate on developing a state of complete trust with one or more animals and the rest will take care of itself.

A New Dawn

With every sunrise we get another shot, another fresh chance to be all we can possibly be. The sun comes with a fresh new start, and the gift of more time. It has a value of incredible promise and hope.

It encourages us to live in pono/balance. Let go of yesterday. Give yourself hope for tomorrow. Live again, and live better – start a new chapter going forward. Be encouraged to live in every moment, and have the attitude that today is it. Enjoy the present, relish the now. You will feel more alive. Live the day to the full and live it as your day. - Ka la hiki Ola

1:26 The Sacred Principles for Healing Yourself and Others

Lomilomi is a healing art practiced by the native Hawaiians. There are many unique forms of this art, traditionally held by each family or O'hana.

Hawaiian Temple Bodywork, Ke Ala Hoku, or Lomilomi Nui (the great massage) is an ancient and distinctive form of lomilomi practiced by the Hawaiian shaman or kahuna in the temples of Hawaii as a sacred rite of passage. This art has been passed down by shamanic teachers committed to sharing their knowledge of this sacred tradition.

I was introduced to Hawaiian Temple Bodywork when I became the recipient of the work at a workshop demonstration. I was so touched by my experience that I moved to Hawaii within six months and devoted the following nine years to studying and practicing this form of healing in Hawaii.

From what I've experienced and observed, this work offers the opportunity for profound personal transformation. The following are several of the principles I've learned and integrated and they have become a guide for me, both as a teacher and practitioner.

The first principle is self-care and honoring yourself as a sacred, unique being. We explore this principle in the workshops, partly through conscious stretching as we open and listen to our bodies physically, and on a feeling and energetic level. We also explore this concept through different exercises: opening our heart center, nurturing ourselves and discovering deeper levels of self-acceptance.

Second, we hold a sacred space for participants, allowing each individual to have their unique experience to discover, acknowledge and embrace all aspects of who they are. The clearer, healthier and more conscious one is, the more one can facilitate wholeness and healing in others. Creating a sacred, safe environment often allows participants to release some of the patterns in their lives that may not be serving them.

Third, we perceive each person as divine and whole in the core of their being. In realizing that there is nothing that is 'wrong' or unworthy in our innate being, there is a tremendous source for self-love, joy, healing and celebration.

Fourth is the principle of movement. Within this sacred space, we begin to move consciously and to learn shamanic exercises to open our body, strengthen our 'mana' or energy level and learn specific techniques that assist us in facilitating transformation and healing for ourselves and others.

Fifth, in an experiential way we explore the principle that answers and healing come from within. While we honor our teachers and the lineages and paradigms we work with, we realize that the ultimate choice, power and responsibility of our lives comes from ourselves and our connection to the Divine.

Sixth is conscious touch. In the workshops we train, explore and deepen our sensitivity to ourselves and others, both physically and energetically. We begin to expand our awareness, integrating the movement and the quality of the work with sacred, conscious touch.

Seventh is the principle of receiving and allowing. Much of the learning in the workshop is in allowing and receiving the work, the touch and the openness from others. As we receive and trust we deepen our connection to ourselves, the earth and the Divine.

Eighth, the principle of facilitation and intention is fundamental to supporting all the other principles. Our intention is to be present and conscious and to create a safe and nurturing space.

Finally, the principle of integration is important for our fast-paced, secular world. Learning to slow down, listen to our inner wisdom and to integrate the experience of the sacredness into our daily lives is essential to our well-being.

Discovering, exploring and sharing these principles of Hawaiian Temple Bodywork in weekend workshops and residential retreats and assisting participants in their growth has been a beautiful and profound gift.

These ancient teachings remind us of our wholeness, our divinity. It's an awakening that allows us to know our unique self, not as a separated individual, but as a connected part of the whole. For me, it is a blessing to travel and share the power and beauty of this work and witness individuals awakening to themselves on such an intimate, soul level. - Tom Cochran and Donna Jason ~ Sacred Lomi

> *"Whoever enters the portal without a guide, will take a hundred years to travel a two day journey."*
>
> Rumi

1:27 The Pathway of the Stars

What is the pathway of the stars? It is our eternal path towards enlightenment. Our first steps may be tentative, but as we proceed, often through many lifetimes, we learn to walk in grace and eventually to be able to free our spirits and dance along the pathway of the stars, to become a stardancer as we move towards enlightenment – now that is a great goal.

All people climb the same mountain of enlightenment. The mountain, however, has many pathways, each with a different view. At the base of the mountain those pathways are wide apart and so are our view points. A person knows and understands only what he sees from his own pathway; as he moves and progresses up the mountain, his view will change, he will see more and understand more. As the seeker gets higher he will begin to notice other people on other paths all heading in the same direction. The middle of the mountain is not as wide as the base and our differences also are not as wide.

Only when we reach the top of the mountain will we see and understand all the views of mankind. But who among us has reached the top of the mountain? Tomorrow, we too will see a different view. We have not finished growing. - **Koko Wills and Pali Jae Lee**

How do we get on to the pathway?

You are already on the path towards enlightenment and have been since time before time. Your journey through many lifetimes has often been hard, you have experienced love and hate, good and bad, childhood and parenthood, and you have been the servant and the master, the murderer and the murdered, the conqueror and the conquered. Only by embracing life completely and experiencing every emotion will your soul have the wisdom of all life within it. Never feel guilty about learning, never feel guilty about wisdom. It's called enlightenment. - **Ramtha**

The portal

Your life's journey has taken you to many places and now you stand on a special stepping stone, for you have arrived at a place of magic. Here the path divides: one appears to enter a lake and the other goes around the lake. The one you can see is a familiar safe route, it will take you on a long route around the lake and eventually to base camp on the mountain to the light. Or will it just circle the lake, bringing you back to where you started, or will it bend another way? My only advice would be to follow your dreams, listen to the feelings within your soul and then embark upon the adventures that your soul urges you to experience. Decide in your heart of hearts what you really enjoy doing, then live a life doing it. I know where you are, because I too have been there.

I looked into the water, the surface glistened under the sun; I could see nothing but experienced a sense of peace. I then decided to take a rest after a long journey and lie down on the soft grass banks. I slowly relaxed into a meditative state as my senses became heightened; I could hear a dew drop from a leaf dropping into the still water somewhere in the distance, I could smell the fresh morning fragrance of the grass and the beautiful flowers – I was glad to be alive.

And then I heard it, the soft sweet sound, the gentle music of the South Pacific, and then a whisper: "Open your eyes my child, look into my world and see anew." As I slowly opened my eyes and took in the scene set before me, I realized that I must have slept all day for it was now dusk, there was a gorgeous sunset on the horizon and then in the twilight I could see her, the shimmering, beautiful essence that is Azura. The lady of the lake, the guardian of the portal between the physical and the spiritual dimensions, she beckoned me to look into the still water; the deep blue water was now crystal clear as it glistened in the moonlight.

As I looked deep into the water a vision appeared. Within the lake is a valley, it was my valley, a valley full of life, full of wonder, there is grass and trees and animals everywhere. To my left was a waterfall running into a large clear pond, from the base of the waterfall rose a beautiful rainbow into the night sky – is it night? As I scanned the water I could see a female dolphin playing joyfully with her calf, there is a family of turtles relaxing in the sun – is it day? It was neither night nor day, just a special moment suspended in time.

As I adjusted to the scene, I noticed that in the distance was a large high mountain with what appeared to be a string of sparkling gems wrapped around its circumference, twisting all the way down from the summit to the base. Then as I adjusted my vision to the far end of the valley, tiny little reflections of starlight could be seen on the grass, and through the forest; they disappeared but then reappeared as they crossed a stone bridge that spanned a rushing river. What was it? It reminded me of fairy dust from a Walt Disney film. Once again it disappeared, hidden from view by a nearby hill, then I could see it. At first it was just one twinkle on the ground, and then two and then three, it was heading in my direction, four, five, six, the light was getting nearer and bigger with every magical glitter. It was now the size of a cheeseburger, and it was growing with each step of awakening light. Then just before it got to me, I lost it behind some reeds and a nearby thicket.

Where did it go? Why had it stopped? As I formulated the questions in my mind, I could hear the soft vibration of Azura; no words were said, but I understood her message:

'You have a choice, stick with the old familiar path or embrace a new future, dare to dream your most incredible dream for anything is possible.'

This is your path, once you step on to it, is the one that only you walk on. No one else can walk your path for you.

When you come to this place of realization, you understand that your life is your practice. When you have been drawn into this connection, wise spirit beings become your teachers and your advisers.

At this point it's not about belief and faith any more. It's about your direct relationship with those spiritual elders who exist in the realm of things hidden; they are poised to help you. And when you have been brought into connection with them, the rest just follows.

To reap the rewards you must pay the price, and the price is high. Nothing less than total commitment to live your life in the light of aloha will result in your desire.

I had been shown the 'pathway of the stars', the stepping stones of life leading towards the source of all knowledge. The choice was clear: I could stay on the old familiar road or I could take a quantum leap through the portal, and have faith that Azura would guide me on a journey through the magical valley of the stars. Only then, and only with 100% commitment, would my next step in life reveal itself in the glitter of the starlite!

"The secret of this magical journey is the concept that we need to achieve a fuller life of love, happiness and spiritual growth. At the core is the wisdom and our job is to unveil it and let it shine through. Life then flows and fear is lost. We can then eagerly accept the challenge life offers us in this particular incarnation.

As we engage with the spirit of aloha and let the light into our own lives, we understand how it can help others, so we share it to the extent that others are willing to consider a new view. Be centered in the light, looking outward without any assumptions of what reality is, open to new experiences of the here and now. From our own center we must look forward, for we cannot perceive in any other way.

These individuals are the seed people who may well determine the shape and orientation of spiritual practice in the western world for much of the next two thousand years."

-Hank Wesselman

"Do not worry if you have built your castle in the air. They are where they should be. Now put the foundations under them."

H.D. Thoreau

1:28 A Glimpse through the Veil

Here are three short experiences of the non-physical; they are presented simply as a point of acknowledgement. For there are many of you who have had similar experiences and don't yet realize the gift you have at your fingertips.

The Dark Man

Has he gone? I was thinking. Should I take another peek? Slowly I summoned up the courage and pulled back the sheet; there was no one there. Quickly I got out of bed and ran into my mum and dad's bedroom. "There is a black man in my bedroom," I said to my startled parents.

"We know," was the reply. My father got up to investigate as I quickly took his place in the warm bed.

Well, they did not find anyone, all the windows and doors were locked and nothing was missing. My parents dismissed the event and told me that it was a bad dream, but I knew differently. I may have been only three or four years old but I knew that the black shadow-like figure at the end of my bed was real, this dark humanoid was there to check on me, to visit me. It meant no harm, that I do know. This was my first real encounter with the spirit world and it would not be the last.

Confirmation of the visit came many years later when my mother, for the only time in her life, referred to that night as the 'visit of evil'. They too had seen the apparition. However, it was far from evil; my overall feeling was one of initial communication and that was to be proved at a later date.

Flying

Have you ever tried to sleep when your knee or any other joint was throbbing? Lying in bed trying to get comfortable and induce a much-needed sleep was not easy with your knee propped up on a pillow. I had just returned home following an operation on my knee and was sleeping in a separate bedroom to my wife, in order to protect my injury and, I think more importantly, to allow her to have a good night's sleep.

My mind was wandering in and out of consciousness when it happened. I was out of my body, facing forward, two feet together and half sitting up and I was flying at full speed through the bedroom door, down the hall to my wife's bedroom. I went straight through the bedroom door, which actually looked more like a hologram than a solid door. I then turned around and looked at my wife from the bottom of the bed, and about six foot in the air I could see the red top she had on The next thing I knew I had traveled at warp speed backwards up through the ceiling, wall and roof and was looking down on my house from about 100 feet in the dark night air.

I had an out of body experience once before when I was a teenager. That time I remember looking down at the sleeping bodies of my brother and me from the ceiling of my bedroom, which at the time felt like a dream. This, however, was different, this was no dream, no hallucination, and this was nothing short of a fully-fledged altered state of expanded awareness. This was more real than my physical 'reality.' In a nanosecond I had taken in details of treetops, hedgerows and noticed a damaged roof tile on the house. I had the overwhelming feeling that I was about to embark on a journey of discovery. We had only been living in the house and neighborhood for a few weeks and at this point I had a conscious thought: I said to myself I must remember how to get back. In a flash I was back in my body. That was over ten years ago and I am still waiting to do that journey. I had, I believe, disconnected myself from whatever energy force that I had engaged with by reinforcing a connection with the physical reality.

By the way, my wife did spend the night in a red top (she had gone to bed after me and I did not know what she had put on; the red top was confirmed in the morning when she brought in a cup of tea). And there was a broken tile on the roof where I had seen it.

Bedrock

I had left New York a few days earlier and my mind was bouncing all over the place. I had been on a quest for 40 years collecting knowledge, bodywork techniques and moulding them into a bodycare system for my own personal use. I was happy to share this with other bodyworkers and massage therapists who were interested in this piece of art. What I did not expect was to link and expand my very personal children's hospice interest with that of my profession. But that is exactly what seemed to be happening, or at least what my pathway seemed to be revealing. There are many good philanthropic organizations out there and I don't really want to be starting yet another one. All of these thoughts were fighting for space as I slowly went into a meditative state. The sun was beating down and the waves were crashing against the rocks. Bermuda really is a beautiful place.

The next thing I noticed was a whirlpool developing in the deep water by the rocks; a dark tunnel seemed to be opening, the bright blue water all the way around it was flashing with light, multi-colors, and sparkling waves. Before I knew it, I was traveling down the tunnel towards a light at the end, but before I got there the water that formed the sides of the tunnel enclosed all around me. It then started to retreat back about six to ten feet to reveal a cave, reddish-brown in color, the walls looked as though they were made from a soft living coral, it was alive with movement, formed but not of form. I sat down on a bed of seaweed and asked if there were any spirit helpers who wished to join me.

Shortly after the cave walls started to reveal non-human faces as though they were carved into the rock, they would fade and re-sculpture themselves. Communication was through thought, and the visual images in the coral/stone cave wall.

I was shown the foundation of the earth being formed from fire, volcanic rock being built upon with layer upon layer of animal and fish bones, plankton to trees. Everything was included, and with each wave-like movement the faces would appear and disappear. The earth is alive, the bedrock, the result of spirit soul memory carved into its very foundation. Therefore the earth is sacred.

How arrogant and ignorant of me in assuming that I was to head some do-good organization. I was simply to be a small flame that as it ceased to exist would leave behind a small sliver of volcanic rock upon which enlightened and enlivened individuals would build the future layers.

I asked for forgiveness, and for the blessing of the earth and earth spirits. I then stated that I would accept the wish of the spirit of the cave. Immediately the walls turned to water, clear blue water cascading down as though it was a waterfall, and then I saw her, there was no mistaking her: Azura in all her glory, or at least the head and flowing hair, her eyes just sparkled and I felt my heart smile.

I was instantly awake and soaking wet, lightening was dancing across the now black sky, the heavens had opened up and Horseshoe Bay was having its own disco show right in the middle of a hot summer's day.

◆ *The O'hana that is Azura was founded by one small light,*
a light of inspiration that encourages self-determination,
self-exploration and spiritual growth through the employment
of aloha energy and spirit to bring smiles and laughter into the
lives of children who are seriously or terminally ill.

As is the human body, so is the cosmic body

As is the human mind, so is the cosmic mind

As is the microcosm, so is the macrocosm.

Ayurveda text

1:29 Questions and Answers

Did the Starlite® bodycare system originate in Hawaii?

The answer to that is no, it is not Hawaiian, its true reflection is oceanic. This is because its origins pre-date the settlement of the Hawaiian Islands; it pre-dates the destruction of Lemuria 'the land of light' that existed in the vast ocean of the Pacific. However, it has Hawaiian influences and derives from the same ancestor seeding, its origins go back deep into oceanic mythology, a mythology that refers to the arrival of starmen from the Pleiades star system as the original light beings 18.5 million years ago. In this period of transformation long ago, in time before time, these light beings became embodied in human form in order to experience life on earth in the physical plane. All across the South Seas, ancient wisdom states that we are not human beings here to have the occasional spiritual experience, but we are spirit beings here to have the human experience, and at the end of that particular incarnation we become disembodied and return to spirit form as light bodies, the physically manifested intelligent energy of the source.

The immediate problem faced by the newly arrived starmen was how to look after and maintain this embodiment, their vehicle and home during their life on the planet earth. Using innate knowledge, a system of care and maintenance was developed that would cover every aspect of body-mind health. This holy and holistic healing system is the origin of Starlite® lomi.

Where was Lemuria?

Some anthropologists can trace this time stream to around 35,000-50,000 years ago. It is believed that Lemuria covered a vast area in what is now the Pacific Ocean; today only the mountain peaks survive as the islands of Hawaii. The population revival started with settlements in Taiwan, Australia and New Guinea.

Oceanic migration started around 5,000 years ago with voyages across the ten million square miles of the Pacific, and settling in new lands. They first came upon the islands of Fiji, Samoa and Tonga. From there they moved eastwards and settled in Tahiti, the Cook Islands and the Marquesas where they stayed for around 1,500 years. The peaceful descendants from the land of Lemuria traveled northward on to Hawaii and the warrior Tahitian descendants traveled south to New Zealand. Eventually, hundreds of years later, the warriors of Tahiti found the peaceful peoples of Hawaii and conquest followed. Even what is accepted today as Hawaiian culture is by definition part of a bigger picture, that of Oceania.

Polynesia is not just a set of tiny island paradises scattered in the Pacific. What some call Micronesia more accurately reflects its size. This area extends from the archipelago of Hawaii in the north to Rapa Nui (Easter Island) in the southeast, and to Aotearoa (New Zealand) in the southwest. Because the islands span the oceans, we refer to their cultures as oceanic.

Where do the names Starlite® and Stardance come from?

Stardance – I was first presented with the name stardance during a shamanic dreamtime experience. I resisted time and time again over a three year period; I protested that you could not call any part of a bodywork therapy stardance, it would not be taken seriously by the complementary therapy or medical communities.

Let's follow accepted protocol and give it a modern or a Hawaiian name was my thinking. Oh, how my ego got in the way of universal intelligence and cosmic energy waves; there was, however, only ever going to be one winner.

During the three year period that followed, work seemed hard, heavy going and frustrating, it felt like we were swimming against the current, using a great amount of energy just to stay afloat. Why stardance, why?

Having been brought up in the western education system and with the western mindset, I need to know in order to accept. This was, on my part, a complete lack of trust of universal intelligence, and indeed even an arrogance to think I should be informed before accepting what is and what will be. Here was a lesson in trust and faith. For me the message from the universe was that shamanic dreamtime is real, time travel and interdimensional travel is real, suspend your 'prove it first' western approach to life and accept that the limitations of your science have not yet evolved sufficiently to understand all of the mysteries of the universe. Only when you yourself remove imposed boundaries, limitations and restrictions, only when you suspend your prejudices and beliefs, will you be free to discover the infinite possibilities available to all entities on this planet.

I had got caught up in the detail and simply forgotten this was not my personal system of bodycare – it belonged to the universe.

A funny thing happened as soon as I accepted the stardance name: my business escalated in many directions that I had not expected or envisioned. It was like the release of energy as you pop a champagne cork from its bottle, we were now definitely going with the flow, a flow that has been gathering momentum ever since. It was here that I learned the concept of cosmic wave riding.

Stardancer – A year or so later, during another dreamtime experience, I was shown a people who existed over 5,000 years ago. They were nomads of the ocean, travelers of the sea, their GPS system was the stars of the night sky, a people whose astral navigational skills where so good, so precise, that it was said they 'danced among the stars'. Another reference was one that relates to the original starmen whose orientation through the universe and the dimensions of spacetime continuum was so accurate and masterful that they were referred to as Stardancers.

The practitioners of this most sacred art were simply known as dancers. *"For they neither seek to wilfully control people or energy. They simply let the life-force flow through uninterrupted by ego and desire, they are inseparable from the wave, their body moving in harmony with the vibration of the surrounding energy, and they become the eye of the storm, a vortex of light energy dancing with joy in a state of grace and gratitude."* - Rima A. Morrell

Some time after I had collected, assembled and polished the techniques of the stardance, I was shown the next level of a far bigger picture, a picture of the Milky Way where my contribution was just one tiny twinkle in a vast ocean of starlight. Today the Stardance™ has evolved to become the quantum core, the one constant element found within the Starlite® bodycare system

What is Azura?

Azura is a voluntary group of people who wish to share the spirit of aloha with the world through the medium of lomilomi. It's a philanthropic O'hana truly reflecting the soul of Hawaii and its people.

A debt of gratitude is owed to the ancestors of the Hawaiian people for the 35,000-year-old survival of the core techniques and philosophy.

There can be no greater gift to the peoples of the earth than that given by the spirit of the islands; there can be no greater way to honor the people of the islands but to live and breathe aloha, in the true expression of the spirit.

Where did the name Azura come from?

Azura is the personification of the powerful energy found at a place of magic, the portal between the physical and spiritual worlds, where night meets day, where life and death merge, a place where all is not what it seems.

This spiritual force, called Azura, is the lady of twilight, a bridge between dimensions; she is a gatekeeper who lives at the interface where two worlds touch. She is the keeper of our dreams.

I was first introduced to Azura during a shamanic dream. This was one of the magical things that happened shortly after I had accepted that I was to use the name Stardance. I found myself in an ocean of fluid energy; it felt like a liquid of sorts charged with sparks of light. Then there she was, directly in from of me; at first she appeared like a glimmering light in female form, a beautiful scene of oscillating energy in various shades of blue and silver with twinkles of light reflecting from her liquid form. She communicated through thought and introduced herself as Azura, the spirit of starlight, in the form of energy that seemed to look like an angel, then a mermaid, then a collection of light, sparks, and wispy form. I understood that she lived in the place where magic happened, the portal between the physical and spiritual dimensions.

In years to come and in years gone by I would see Azura on many occasions, in her angelic mermaid form in the spiritual dimension and in the form of a dolphin in the physical world. She would appear just at sunset or during the time of the moonshadow. But, that's another story...

STOP PRESS

Hoku

Once again I have been shaken to the core. The manuscript for this book has just been edited and the printing press is ready to go, then bam!

For three weeks now I have been on an emotional roller-coaster, with nightly visits from the aumakua who are ancestral **guardian spirits keepers of the knowledge. I feel battered, black and blue,** it's as though I have been trapped in the surf rolling over and over having my flesh stripped away as my body is pushed and pulled against the black lava rocks, finally my bones are broken and all that is left is the beating heart of my core, the light of my soul. I surrender totally to the universal force and accept my fate, whatever that may be. As I do so, I feel free and at one with the eternal beauty of creation. Then the curtain of the night opens, just enough to let in a single ray of light healing energy from the stars, in this light I can see four symbols twisting and rolling towards me, the symbols are letters and a game of scrabble unfolds before my eyes, eventually they settle resting gently in my hand and the word 'Hoku' appears. I don't know the meaning of the word but I am immediately overcome by a great sense of gratitude and tears of delight roll from my eyes which are sparkling with the energy of the divine. I have just received a very precious gift wrapped in the love of aloha, and the permission to use a Hawaiian word and that word is Hoku (star). In honour and gratitude to the ancestral beings of light it is my privilege to present Hoku® lomi (stardance) as the beating heart of the starlite® system.

1:30 Our Deepest Fear

The following is a beautiful expression and acceptance of our spirit being, it is often wrongly attributed to Nelson Mandela and his acceptance speech. However, I am sure that Marianne Williamson will agree it is a great reflection of his spirit.

"Our deepest fear is not that we are inadequate. Our deepest fear is that we are powerful beyond measure. It is our light, not our darkness, that most frightens us. We ask ourselves: Who am I to be brilliant, gorgeous, talented, and fabulous? Actually, who are you not to be? You are a child of the Divine. Your playing small doesn't serve the world. There's nothing enlightened about shrinking so that other people won't feel insecure around you. We are all meant to shine, as children do. We are born to make manifest the glory of the divine spirit that is within us. It's not just in some of us, it's in everyone. And as we let our own light shine, we unconsciously give other people permission to do the same. As we are liberated from our own fear, our presence automatically liberates others."

- Marianne Williamson

1:31 The Tree of Life

◆ *A sacred esoteric knowledge found in the akashic records of the mystical cosmic and collective consciousness has been encoded in the non-physical plane of existence and given as a precious gift to the peoples of the blue planet.*

Pre-history:

◆ *Ancient oceanic knowledge proclaims that 'starmen, beings of light' came into our physical dimension and settled on earth approximately 18 million years ago.*

◆ *We are not human beings here to have a spiritual experience; we are embodied spirit beings here to have the human experience.*

◆ *There existed a land called Lemuria 'the land of light' approximately 36,000 years ago.*

◆ *Here they developed a system of care and healing for their new physical embodiment.*

◆ *This was an ancient lomilomi bodycare system.*

◆ *Lomilomi was the healing tree of life for the oceanic people.*

◆ *Oceanic lomilomi included: massage; cleansing; hot and cold therapy; energy work; healing plants; stone and crystals therapy; health education; counselling; philosophy; bone setting; diet; physical therapy; skeletal manipulation; exercise; martial arts.*

◆ *They lived gracefully with aloha.*

◆ *They had direct contact with the community of light, the source guardians.*

◆ *They were one with the loving spirit and enveloped the vitality of goodness, light and love.*

◆ *They were known as the people of secret power.*

◆ *They had a unique philosophy for successful living.*

◆ *Called 'the way of the sacred light' founded on universal love.*

◆ *The tree of life was uprooted when their continent was destroyed in a single night.*

◆ *Few of the original starmen survived; those who did became nomads on a vast new ocean. They became the oceanic people.*

◆ *Master navigators of the ocean, it was said that like their ancestors they 'danced with the stars'.*

◆ *Around 3500BC the Proto-Polynesian people started to settle on various islands, constantly moving east away from warring tribes.*

◆ *Around 1500BC they eventually settled on the Marquesas Islands.*

◆ *They stayed for around 2000 years. Many Hawaiian families can trace their family line back to 800BC.*

- *There followed an idyllic time of love, peace and happiness.*

- *About 650AD after being discovered by warrior nations they left and traveled 1800 miles north across the vast ocean, following a star, until they reached the Island of Molokai.*

- *The people spread out to Lanai, Kauai, Maui, and Hawaii.*

- *On these islands they planted their own variations of the tree of life, each with a new lineage.*

- *Life was beautiful.*

- *All lived in harmony.*

- *Around 1100AD Hawaii was invaded by warriors from Tahiti who installed the order of Ku.*

- *The invaders tried to destroy the original teachings; they hunted and killed the priest.*

- *The ancient ones hid the original teachings in chants and in the Hula dance.*

- *The invaders unwittingly adopted the chants and the Huna.*

- *In 1778 Captain James Cook lands in Hawaii.*

- *In 1820 when the missionaries arrived from Boston they set about saving the souls of the heathens.*

- *It was outlawed to practice massage Huna, and the penalty was prison.*

- *Now for a second time the secret knowledge was buried to a deeper level.*

- *Priests and kahunas became aunties and uncles.*

- *1850 Hawaiian-American Treaty.*

- *1893 Hawaii surrenders to US.*

- *1900 Hawaii becomes US Territory.*

- *Native population reduced from 300,000+ in 1778 to 30,000 in 1900 due to traders diseases.*

- *1972 Sorcery law lifted (imprisonment from Lomi massage practice).*

- *1979 US law changed allowing native healers to practice.*

- *This was followed by a re-growth.*

- *But natives were not interested, they had adopted the easier modern lifestyle.*

- *Skills and knowledge had been lost and only a few knew the secrets.*

- *Some would have to go back, return to the origins of lomilomi buried deep in antiquity, long before any lineage began.*

- *To keep lomilomi and Huna alive and to ultimately return it to its former glory, the secret and aloha spirit had to be shared with the world.*

- *Native kahunas taught lomilomi massage.*

- *They shared the ancient knowledge now called Huna.*

- *First to a few chosen spirits with island lineage and connections.*

- *They in turn spread the word around the world.*

- *But in the sharing of the knowledge came the ever present danger of dilution.*

- *The tree of life is starting to grow again, this time its mission is to offer the fruit of aloha to all the peoples of the blue planet.*

Part Two

STARLiTE
The Secret Lomi

Discovering the sacred touch of aloha

Part Two

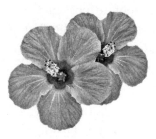

Not all knowledge is found in one school...

2:32 About the Rainbow Course

From the very first module you will be introduced to the mystical techniques that make up the central core of this amazing energy bodycare system and the shamanic principles found within Huna. You will learn how to embrace spiritual energy and apply it to loving touch healing. You will learn the art of oceanic Laulima, an ancient energy work with special healing powers. Step by step, you will be introduced to aloha touch and active release techniques that make up the central core of this beautiful bodycare system.

You will learn basic to advanced techniques of soft tissue mobilization, how to increase joint range of motion, improve skeletal alignment and anatomical balance of the body. You will learn how to actively release stress and tension, activate the hormonal and chemical interchange in the body and bring about improved health and well-being.

You will learn how to weave loving energy from the cosmos 'sparks of light' into these beautifully choreographed techniques, creating a magical shamanic dance, infused with the spirit of aloha.

You will explore the infinite possibilities of this powerful and potentially life-changing esoteric healing therapy, learn to ride cosmic waves and experience a multidimensional universe where shamanism and quantum physics merge in an ocean of pure potentiality.

This course is lomilomi in its purest form – 'spirit touching spirit'. It is an adventure in discovering and loving your emotional body, the sharing of aloha, love, caring, and compassion. You will be able to experience the magic of the oceanic people and have a foundation for the 'adventure of a lifetime'.

> *"I don't massage, I reset.*
> *It's called body alignment."*
>
> Papa Kalua Kaiahua

Starlite® Lomi Bodycare System brings together a synthesis of techniques and a touch of magic. It is a fusion of ancient wisdom, modern knowledge and the spirit of aloha. This creates a faculty of inner awareness to promote a drastic jump, a quantum leap, in the healing mechanism. A new dawn is rising for this most sacred of bodycare systems.

2:33 Seven Stages of Starlite Treatment

A Starlite® bodycare session can be divided into seven stages or steps:

- ◆ *Preparation*
- ◆ *Pule*
- ◆ *Alo~Ha Breath*
- ◆ *Hoku (stardance)*
- ◆ *Bone Washing*
- ◆ *Laulima*
- ◆ *Wave Break*

Stage One ~ *Preparation*

A Starlite® session starts when a person calls to make an appointment, for they have set their intention and activated a connection; this in turn activates subtle healing forces. They will receive an active preparation meditation, this can often cause shifts in ordinary reality as precursory energies awaken and begin circulating. We call this the twilight period, a portal of potential standing between the dark of night and the light of day.

It's a period when strange magical things can occur and people should take notice of special dreams or new insights.

Before leaving home they should shower and shave any areas that they normally do. Any stubble will feel uncomfortable to both giver and receiver.

When they are en route to our healing space for their appointment they enter a more pronounced period, a portal of opportunity, a period that we refer to as sunrise. They can benefit enormously by turning off any distractions, engaging in meditative breathing, and focusing their attention on the joy of the journey, which is not always easy, but has great rewards if you can achieve it.

The therapist must set a sacred space (Halau), a comfort zone for healing and learning. He or she should make sure that the space is clean and clear, with the right atmosphere, temperature and music set, then finally surround it with an orchid curtain. They should also adopt an attitude that is clean and positive in mind, body and spirit. - **Shamanic Reiki**

Stage Two ~ *Pule*

Set clear intentions, for as we call for spirit you will automatically enter in the Halau, the sacred space.

Prayer belongs in lomilomi, it is our connection to divine light, universal energy. Over time it has been transformed from traditional prayer to Christian prayer, and recently once again transformed by modern understanding of energy and quantum physics into 'wilful, conscious intent'.

"Directed consciousness is the power that makes magic happen. Great focus brings great power. Every society on earth prays, and what else is prayer but directed consciousness that sets up a link with the sacred?" - Rima A. Morrell

Pule is the switch that turns on the light. *"This transition does not diminish the authenticity of modern lomilomi; it merely demonstrates how the healing arts can change with times."* - Robert Noah Calvert

Stage Three ~ *Ha Breath*

The real conduit of healing, the core, is in using breath as medicine. If pule is the switch then the Ha Breath is the flow of energy that raises the vibration to a level for healing.

"Breath is timeless, as is the wind of time. Nothing is permanent, thus providing the opportunity for change and adjustment." - Kahu Abraham Kawai'i

All life on earth is based in wavelengths of energy called electromagnetic radiation. Within this spectrum of visible light, we perceive different 'vibrations' of light, and each of us attracts things into our lives according to our own 'vibration of light'. Using Ha Breath we intend to raise the vibration of the receiver to the level of healing light.

For Hawaiians, two higher emotions/vibrations are the easiest sources for healing:

◆ *Gratitude: communion through gratitude.*

◆ *Laughter: the purest form of communication and communion with spirit.*

Stage Four ~ *Hoku (stardance)*

Using a beautifully choreographed dance, the practitioner gracefully and systematically works their way through the soft tissue of the body. In an ebb and flow of cosmic waves, blocked energy is released, and fresh new light energy introduced. The practitioner alternates between active soft tissue release techniques (ART) and energy enhancement techniques (ATT); the result is a 'magical dance of the tissues'.

Stage Five ~ *Bone Washing*

The finishing touches start with bone washing and the cleaning of the aura, by pulling the old energy, emotions, aches and pains out through the extremities and throwing them away.

Stage Six ~ *Laulima*

Once the old energy has been removed, Laulima may be used to keep open the connection to the universal source of energy and the body's own energy circuitry systems. A constant flow of cosmic waves carrying life-enhancing energy cascades through the body. 'From spirit to me, from me to you, from you to spirit, the circle is complete.'

This is a giving time, it's grace-receiving gratitude.

Often during this stage the receiver may experience a 'starburst' moment, a feeling of infinite space, or a flash of sudden awareness, sometimes called a satori moment.

Grace: (complete and unconditional love)

"Grace is the inalienable right of all beings to receive the light of spirit, the inalienable source of all healing. From the power of spirit comes this completely unconditional love, which heals and propels support. Grace is absolutely free and is not something that can be taken away from you. When grace appears in the consciousness the natural response is gratitude. Gratitude is the action linking the grace to us. Grace connects and deepens the channel of gratitude." - Harry Uhane Jim

Stage Seven ~ *Wave Break*

Aka is the Hawaiian Huna word for the energy substance which surrounds us and connects us to each other; it is how information and life force and energy travel. All contact, whether in the physical or on another level, involves the exchange of threads of Aka material or 'sticky' energy waves.

In order to keep a professional distance between the giver and the receiver it is important that any Aka energy connection is cut on completion thus separating or breaking your energy waves from theirs.

This method is very simple and is done in a loving act of gratitude, sending both thanks (Mahalo) and blessings to both spirit and receiver.

The final touch on the receiver should be on their shoulders. Bring your hands up to the Kanku position, then thank the spirit for attending the session with a simple Mahalo and blessings, sharply separate your hands. Breathe in deeply and at the same time bring your arms down and around so that the palms are facing the ground. Do this while sending love, gratitude and blessings through the cords to the receiver. Disconnect by sharply throwing any unwanted or blended energy to the ground, with the wish that it is used for the greater good.

2:34 Rainbow Course Overview

The Rainbow Course relates specifically to the Stardance™ stage of a Starlite® treatment session.

The Stardance™ is probably the most technically advanced lomilomi bodycare procedure in the world.

It is a specially selected collection of soft tissue mobilization techniques that have been woven into a beautifully choreographed dance.

The practitioner alternates between energy enhancing aloha touch and active release soft tissue techniques woven into a beautifully choreographed dance. She/he gracefully and systematically surfs through the cosmic waves of concentrated vibrated energy that comprise the human body.

The aim is to bring the physical (musculoskeletal) and energetic body back towards pono (balance) allowing the body to work at its maximum potential, within its own set of circumstances. To achieve this, the practitioner looks to find and actively release blocked energy within the body tissues, often associated with Somatic Dysfunction and/or Dysponesis. When the practitioner finds a blockage of condensed energy within the musculoskeletal system, she/he will use a combination of ART techniques specially designed for each body part and ATT techniques to raise the vibration of the blockage. This will result in a 'magical dance of the tissues' releasing the blocked energy and creating space within the tissue.

> *"Once new space has been created, you the giver direct the force of gratitude (aloha spirit) from your heart to the body of the receiver. When gratitude is released, it sends signals to the entire body to heal whatever the wounds may be, and their body innately knows how to take care of itself."* - Harry Uhane Jim

> *"The ultimate goal of the dance is to weave a beautiful rainbow of healing light."* - Rima A. Morrell

Active Release Techniques:

◆ *ART techniques enable the practitioner to work at the interface of energy and structure.*

◆ *Allow a little pocket of powerful kinetic energy to be directed into the body at a precise place and angle to maximize the energy's encouragement of the innate response.*

◆ *The intention behind all ART techniques is to reduce tension in the musculoskeletal system by releasing blocked energy, and thus nourish the body's innate repair mechanism by encouraging a state of balanced posture and ease.*

◆ *Allow the therapist to work with the receiver, encouraging universal intelligence and the body's own innate repair system to work at an optimum.*

Somatic Dysfunction:

◆ *Defined as impaired or altered function of related components of the somatic (body framework) system, skeletal, arthrodial, and myofascial structures and related vascular, lymphatic, and neural elements (somatic dysfunction is a comprehensive term).*

◆ *Allows for the use of various therapeutic techniques to maximize the healing potential of the dysfunctional element.*
- Leon Chaitow

Dysponesis:

◆ *A reversible physiopathological state consisting of unnoticed, misdirected, neurophysiological reactions to various agents (environmental, body sensations, emotions and thoughts) and the repercussions of these reactions throughout the organism.*

◆ *These errors in energy expenditure, which are capable of producing functional disorders, consist mainly of covert errors in action potential output, from motor and premotor areas of the cortex and the consequences of that output.*

◆ *Spinal dysponesis – a condition of one or more spinal segments that have lost their ability to move freely or completely throughout their range of rotation that physically interfere with the spinal cord and/or spinal nerves and their function.* - Dr. Jay Holder

Bones as soft tissue:

◆ *"Because bodyworkers become so accustomed to studying synthetic or 'dead' osseous structures it is easy to forget that living bone is really just another soft connective tissue much* like ligament and cartilage. The bones of the body have a rich blood supply with crystals of hydroxyapatite deposited in them for strength and stability but at the same time they are blessed with enough flexibility to allow them to absorb shock and endure injury.

◆ Living bone is viscoelastic. It responds to load by bone deformation, much like fascia responds to load by plastic deformity. Skeletal muscles move bones and at the end range of movement (physiologic barrier), the ligaments protect the joint by restraining further motion. In an attempt to understand the subtle workings of the osseous structures, the modern manual therapist must not be afraid to palpate and mobilize the skeletal system. The more the therapist palpates and evaluates the bony structures of their clients' bodies, the clearer the relationship of the myofascial and skeletal systems becomes and the more holistic and therapeutic the intervention." - Eric Dalton

Quantum:

◆ The quantum is the minimum amount of physical entity involved in an interaction.

◆ The indivisible unit in which waves may be emitted or absorbed. (Dr Stephen Hawking)

◆ In layman's terms, it is a building block which cannot be broken down into anything smaller. It uses a systematic and holistic treatment flow where everything gets checked in order and nothing gets forgotten, but each treatment still remains individual. The Stardance™ module is the quantum unit found within the Starlite® bodycare system and is the only element that stays constant, it is the nucleus around which the other elements resonate.

Cosmic wave:

◆ A cosmic wave is a discontinuous movement, a wave of vibration, of possibility in a universal ocean of pure potentiality. They are powerful accelerated energy waves of expanded consciousness weaving the fabric of space and time.

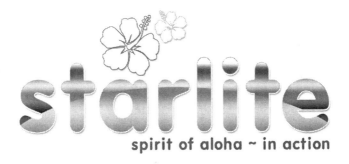

spirit of aloha ~ in action

Starlite® ~ 'rainbow course'

Course consists of soft tissue active release techniques used in the stardance:

Red module
Treatment area: Head, neck and face.

Includes 'sparkle' – aloha~lomi face massage.

Certificated~ stand alone or can be included in treatment.

Orange module
Treatment area: The feet.

Includes lomi feet massage.

Certificated~ stand alone or can be included in treatment.

Yellow module
Treatment area: Anterior lower limb.

Green module
Treatment area: Keystone ~ the pelvis and anterior torso.

Blue module
Treatment area: Hand and upper limb.

Indigo module
Treatment area: Superficial back and lower limb.

Violet module
Treatment area: Deep back and spinal support muscles.

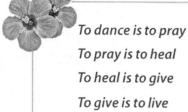

To dance is to pray
To pray is to heal
To heal is to give
To give is to live

2:35 Seven Secrets of the Stardance™

The concept of holism and the need to acknowledge the spirit as much as the body goes deep back into oceanic philosophy.

This holistic approach, caring for the whole person – mind, body and spirit – is one of the factors that draws people to most complementary therapies as opposed to orthodox medical care.

1 Connection
cosmic connection through wilful conscious intention to the power of the universe is the thermodynamic driving force.

2 Expression
of universal energy~ channel of energy.

3 Expansion
of space, creating space in the body to accommodate energy.

4 Quantum
minimum required, for mobilization of all joints and soft tissue.

5 Intervention
introduction of advanced ART techniques by therapist.

6 Integration
of technique, knowledge and energy.

7 Awakening
an awakening of the body to a new day, a new dawn.

Result = Gratitude

"Every human, regardless of race, sex or spiritual belief, has the incredible capacity to accomplish far beyond what they think their limits are."

Source unknown

2:36 White Course overview

"The art is concealed in the art."

Koko

Satori:

A Japanese term that roughly translates into individual enlightenment, or a sudden flash of awareness, a consciousness of an undreamed new truth. Satori is also seen as an intuitive experience. The feeling of satori is that of infinite space.

The only way that one can 'attain' satori is through personal experience.

Starburst:

Often mind, body and spirit systems experience an increase of energy accepted as a benefit of the treatment.

However, it's only when the entire 'body galaxy' experiences the loving and magical power of the universe in an abnormally high explosion of energy (an orgasmic power trip that can restore and revitalize your energy – it is direct spirit-to-spirit link, a lightning bolt of power, full of light and energy) that it can be described as a starburst. A truly unique and mind-blowing experience.

A starburst is the ultimate experience of this sacred bodycare system. When both giver and receiver have moved beyond therapy and have become totally immersed in the 'dance of the stars' as grace and aloha dance to their own tune through the instrument that is the human body.

"When my partner put his hand on my heart, I felt like a galaxy burst open and streamed out light. That light was powerful, emotional. It was blessed, blessed gratitude.

In a second, literally, the grief flies out. I feel wave after wave of release. Rushes of energy pour through my heart and out the top of my head, and then I feel an enormous, cosmic-size gratitude and brilliance. It is a huge gratitude wave."

- Garnette Arledge

Esoteric studies

A sacred esoteric knowledge found in the akashic records of the mystical cosmic and collective consciousness has been encoded in the non-physical plane of existence and given as a precious gift, to the peoples of the blue planet.

Any training in esoteric studies should increase positive character traits in the initiate; above all, it should bring increasing balance of the mind and over time tunes the pupil to higher and higher levels of vibration. - Tad James

Here the earth is viewed as a divine school of esoteric studies – the University of Life, and daily life as the classroom for gaining experience, knowledge and growth.

When finished with the learning process you move to a new level of training. There is no one other than you who has the power to give you initiation or the power to refuse it to you; as soon as you are ready for initiation you claim it by right.

Laulima energy work may be required to open up the energy circuitry so that energy can flow more easily. 'As she spoke, the energy flowed out in waves from her. It was as if she had actually plugged into a source of energy, and was transmitting it out in circles.'

Let go of the notion 'I am only human'; you are human, but not only human. Remember who you are, you are a being of light – that is your heritage.

The science that is now called Huna we believe to be as old as 35,000 years and is part of the original teachings of the peoples of the earth and centered in Hawaii on a continent that no longer exists. - Tad James

"When humanity embraces spirit, a cascade of aloha will rain down upon the earth ~ A Rainbow Cascade."

Koko

2:37 Rainbow Energy

Rainbow medicine (color energy). Pure white light contains the whole spectrum of color and when reflected through water it will display a beautiful rainbow of cascading light energy.

Starlite® lomi works by tuning into the vibration of the universe and channeling cosmic energy waves through spacetime continuum into an embodiment here in the physical dimension.

Cosmic energy is simply light energy resonating at various wavelengths. Each wavelength will have a slightly different vibration and be seen in the physical world as a different color.

For the majority of the time, a stardancer will find that she/he is channeling pure white light directly from the source. However, there are times when a receiver will require a rebalancing of a specific energy vibration and the color of that wave will become apparent to those with eyes that can see through the veil of the physical realm. *"Real vision is seeing the invisible."* - Jonathan Swift

Color and bodywork

All life on earth is based in wavelengths of energy called electromagnetic radiation. What we experience as visible light is simply a tiny portion of this continuum. Electromagnetic radiation of this wavelength activates the nerve cells in our eyes.

Within this spectrum of visible light, we perceive different 'vibrations' of light. We call the visible quality of differentiation of vibration 'color.' We perceive different colors according to their vibration and name them accordingly: red, blue, and yellow. These colors don't exist in the world on their own – they are simply names for light waves of different energy and frequency. - **Principles of Visual Perception by Carolyn Bloomer**

Breathe in the Rainbow

This is a lovely and very helpful exercise to encourage a balance of all the seven main chakra colors for our well-being.

Stand with feet slightly apart and arms by your side, relaxed, with palms turned to the front. Relax the shoulders, and concentrate on your breathing, consciously relaxing all of your body from the top of your head to the tips of your toes. Breathe in deeply through the nose, holding for a few moments and then breathe out through the mouth. As you breathe out, imagine expelling all the stress, negativity and toxins from your body. If you can do this exercise outside all the better, and, weather permitting, stand on grass with bare feet.

Affirmations, either spoken out loud or as a concentrated thought, can be helpful too to help us focus and stop our minds from wandering. For example, red is the color of courage and strength. We could say to ourselves: the energy of red fills my body and I have the strength and courage to move forward along my life's path. It doesn't matter how we word our affirmations – they will be unique to each individual – but remember the positive aspects of the colors and make sure your statements are positive.

Choose the color that has the positive aspect that you require on this occasion and use this still-point meditation technique to re-balance your being. Remember that white contains all the colors of the rainbow and is considered a sacred color.

"Energy Flows ~ where attention goes."

Serge Kahili King

2:38 Energy Flows

How to focus your attention

Exercise:

Take a deep breath and exhale slowly. Now hold out your right hand, palm facing you, with your arm relaxed. Pay close attention to your hand. Observe its size and shape. Look at the skin color. Now see all the lines on the palm of your hand. Focus your attention on them so intently that you could even draw them on a piece of paper.

Imagine there is a dial on your palm that can measure the intensity of your concentration. The highest number on that dial is seven, and the needle is now at three. As your concentrated attention becomes more intense, the needle moves to four. Now let's move it up to five as you feel how the intensity of your concentration increases. Now imagine moving it to six. Now go to the highest number on the dial, seven, and feel the sharp focus of your attention. Hold that focus for one minute.

Now relax your hand, but leave it in front of you, and relax your focus.

Put out your other hand. Do you see or feel any difference between the two hands?

You may have noticed heat, tingling, or a change of color, size or plumpness in the hand on which you focused your attention.

These effects are the result of a biological energy flow following the path between your mind and the object of your concentrated awareness. - Kala H. Kos

Wherever you direct your attention, your energy flows. Your sustained, focused attention channels the energy of the universe into manifesting the equivalent of what you are focusing on.

- Serge Kahili King

"The mind is like a parachute, it doesn't work if it isn't open."

Frank Zappa

2:39 Energy in physical therapy

Energy can be understood at many levels. At the physical level we see energy and structure. Structure is seen as solid matter and energy is found in the elements such as wind, fire, water, light and even electricity. Even at this basic level there is an acceptance of spiritual energy.

The healing arts tend to operate at a level far removed from this model. At this level of working, universal energy can be accessed by a therapist/practitioner/guide and directed/transferred/conducted into structure/a human body for the benefit of the receiver. Most energy systems work at this level; the chakra and meridian systems identify with the concept of channeling energy into structure/body, they show energy running through the body in a particular pattern and talk about the interface of energy and structure. In shamanism what we see as structure is seen as having its own spirit, its own life force.

Practitioners of Starlite® lomi bodycare are able to enter the shamanic world and work at the next level of understanding – a level where solidity of matter and structure is just an illusion. Their understanding is that everything is energy; structure and matter are nothing more than concentrated vibrated energy, resonating at a deep slow vibration, and universal healing energy being channeled vibrates at a higher and faster frequency. When the two meet there is an initial separation of energy waves, then comes the integration. Rivers of energy flow through the body as identified by the chakra and meridian systems, but at the river banks there is a natural blending as two become one. The newly introduced wave of healing energy slowly weaves its way through the web of the more densely concentrated energy, just as water from a river will slowly penetrate and bring life to the earth surrounding the river. At this level we are no longer working with energy and structure, just energy in all its glory.

> *A little wave laps up from the ocean's surface, becoming an incident in the space-time world.*
>
> *The whole ocean remains behind, a vast, silent reservoir of possibilities, of waves not yet born…*
>
> Deepak Chopra

2:40 Cosmic wave

What is a cosmic wave?

A cosmic wave is a discontinuous movement, a wave of vibration, of possibility in a universal ocean of pure potentiality. They are powerful accelerated energy waves of expanded consciousness weaving the fabric of space and time.

The flow of life is nothing other than the harmonious interaction of all the elements and forces that structure the field of existence.

Life is the eternal dance of consciousness that expresses itself as the dynamic exchange of impulses of intelligence between microcosm and macrocosm, between the human body and the universal body, between the human mind and the cosmic mind. - Barbara Chang

Lomilomi is an ancient art, healing separation through the touch of aloha and divine love.

It is the ultimate dance, an intimate loving treatment and a rite of passage...

2:41 Filters

We are spirit embodied in human form; along with the physical form comes a brain which is connected by our sensory systems, and our sensory systems have their own limitations. The eyes can only see a very small part of the spectrum of light, the whole spectrum of light is itself a collection of universal energy waves, and we can only tune into a small part of that universal knowledge. The same could be said of the sound wave spectrum. Again, we have limited access; dogs, for instance, have greater hearing abilities than us – once again we can only tune into a small part of the available universal knowledge. We have an extra sensory system that is under-used and underdeveloped, not because we have limited access, but because we impose our own limitations of mind growth on ourselves. If we are to grow as individuals and as a species, we need to explore the human mind and its unlimited potential. As we start to grow, in mind and spirit, we will connect to the next level of universal knowledge, and a world of wonders will open up to us.

It is here beyond the veil that we will find the future of the healing arts and access to a purity of healing energy.

Healing energy is like water, it is life giving and life saving. However contaminated, water can be life taking and life ending. Ask yourself, are you contaminating your life giving water (life force energy) with unclean filters?

Our understanding of channeling healing energy is thus:

Healing energy:

We originate from universal life force energy and by regular practice we come to understand that we are energy – separate only by illusion. We can connect to this energy for the purpose of channeling healing energy for the benefit of others.

How to do this?

Place your hands on to the receiver and divine healing energy will flow to wherever it will do most good, directed innately by the intelligence of the energy itself.

Are we involved?

A giver is nothing more than a hollow reed, allowing the energy to pass through their own body into that of the receiver. It is a completely egoless action.

Conditions:

Divine healing energy must be transmitted with a loving heart and not from the head.

Growth:

The pure loving light of aloha reveals itself to you as you experience it. And here's the thing! As you use the energy, you multiply it, sending even more loving energy back into the universe.

Filters:

This is a very general understanding of using healing energy; it may vary in detail as found in the different forms of the healing arts, but as a general exercise it is universal. The first two parts – what is healing energy and how to use it – are covered in detail within this book.

We have within us two sets of filters: natural and manmade. Nature's filters are positive and protect us from overload. Total knowledge of the universe may just overload our minds, minds that can only handle 60,000-80,000 thoughts a day. Experts have estimated that our nervous system, through our five senses, is bombarded by two million bits of data each second of the day. We can only digest 126 bits of that data, which boils down to seven (plus or minus two) manageable chunks each second. Our filters take out the rest of the data by deleting, distorting and generalizing information. That's a lot of data to get rid of. No wonder two people remember the same event differently.

The following statement is important because it contains a secret, a pocket of knowledge hidden between the words.

> *'Divine healing energy must be transmitted with a loving heart and not from the head. A giver is nothing more than a hollow reed, allowing the energy to pass through their own body into that of the receiver. It is a completely egoless action.'*
>
> - Shamanic Reiki

First of all, our understanding is that the giver 'is nothing more than a hollow reed, allowing the energy to pass through their own body into that of the receiver'. As we know that the energy in question is 'divine healing energy' then it stands to reason that if we were just a hollow reed and divine energy passed through that reed, the pure healing energy would reach the receiver and miracles would happen every day, as identified in various holy books.

How many of us complementary therapists can claim to have witnessed miracles on a daily basis as our clients rise from the bench cured from all ills?

The logical conclusion is that if divine energy is entering the top of the reed, then something is happening to change its purity as it travels through the reed.

The answer may be found in the rest of the statements. 'It is a completely egoless action' or at least it should be, and 'this energy must be transmitted with a loving heart and not from the head'. Why? Because the head contains all of our filters which may defuse the light, contaminate the water, or become diffused and contaminate the purity of the healing energy. This would explain why two therapists who have had the some training, and access the same universal power, will get different results.

The truth is we are not a hollow reed, but a permeable reed full of filters, filters of varying thicknesses. Those filters are made up of our past experiences, our beliefs, our values, our memories, our religions, our thoughts, our moods, our emotions, and our perception of the world. And each of us has a different set of filters even if we come from the same family or practice the same healing art.

These filters will manifest themselves as thoughts, and thoughts become emotions, emotions will produce a chemical release in the body, that chemical release changes the vibration of the body's energy, the permeable reed allows for the transfer of chemicals and hormones in the form of energy waves, thus contaminating the healing energy being channeled, resulting in a change of the quality of your touch and a dilution of the healing energy.

"Every second of every day external events are impacting on our thoughts. Those events enter our nervous system after going through our personal filters." - Lindsey Agness

Improvement:
Now that we understand the impurity of our human embodiment can and does affect the light we are trying to assist, we can take steps to reduce and/or remove some of these filters, safe in the knowledge that every small reduction results in improvement of the self, and improvement as a healing artist. As we grow in our art, the purity of the light begins to shine through with magical results.

Future growth:
'Divine healing energy must be transmitted with a loving heart.'

We should not influence or affect the purity of light energy that is working through us. In order to do things we should aim to reduce or remove each filter in turn.

Probably the biggest and most difficult filter to reduce or remove is the one marked 'Love yourself'. We need to remove the ego of the mind and body, but love with all our being the spirit within, which originates from the Divine.

Before you can truly love someone else, you have to learn to love yourself, accept yourself for the beautiful loving entity that you are. Accept your greatness, your authenticity, apologize to no one for being you, be yourself, love yourself and then radiate that love to others in the world.

> *"The only way we can be great to ourselves is not what we do with our bodies, but what we do to our minds."* - Ramtha

> *"Bring imagination into a quantum fury... a dream that sets its sights above the mundane and the mediocrity of life. That everyone can set their sights therein. Then we are no longer hated and despised, but we have done the one most excellent virtue – we have saved ourselves through simply applying our most excellent eternal ability and that is that we are as god (grace of divinity), and we call out of inertness the wind-sprayed particles of chaos and we freeze them for a momentary reality, in which all predecessors and all successors agree upon, and now we have tangibility of mass... but we brought it out of nothing and how could we ever be nothing? It is only out of nothing that we have our being. But our being we do have, and we are ambitious spirits."* - Ramtha

Change our attitude and we will change from the inside out...

2:42 Removing Filters and Learn to Love Yourself

Before you can truly love someone else... you have to learn to love yourself, accept yourself for the beautiful loving entity that you are. Accept your greatness, your authenticity, apologize to no one for being you, be yourself, love yourself and then radiate that love to others in the world.

Often this is the biggest filter to reduce or remove. It is not the remit of this book to be a comprehensive teaching manual; it's more of a brochure, a glimpse of what can be. It's your life's path and no one can walk it for you, and no one can learn for you.

Baby steps:

Think of your closest friend or family member, now imagine stepping into their body and seeing through their eyes. Look at yourself, and ask yourself, What do I see? Do you see someone who criticizes and puts themselves down? Who feels bad about their body? Who thinks that they don't deserve to be loved? Make a list of your feelings.

Now remember that 'you are what you think'. But no matter how strongly you believe something, it does not make it true.

If you keep telling yourself that you don't deserve to be loved, you will believe it. As Confucius said: "Every journey begins with the first step." The first step towards learning to love you is a powerful one.

Stop thinking negative thoughts!

> *"The most common blocks are the negative attitudes that a lot of people carry around all the time. In order to become healed, a person has to throw out hatred, envy, jealousy, and other destructive attitudes and feelings. Although such factors start within the mind, they quickly manifest in the body, becoming a stiff neck, a sluggish liver, cancer, or other illness. I believe that all genuine healing addresses the problem of unblocking negative energy in one way or another."* - Sun Bear

We are not asking you to do positive thinking (although that is a very good habit), just stop doing negative thinking, and things will start to change.

Now answer the next three questions truthfully:

1 *How many people have **you** said "I love you" to?*
   (and really meant it)

2 *How many people have said "I love you" **to you?***
   (and really meant it)

3 *How many times have you used this magical word*
   and said "I love you" to yourself?

- Rhonda Britten

Shocked? If so, do the following exercise:

When you wake up in the morning, look in the mirror, look into your eyes, you may be drawn to one in particular. Look deep into your eyes, for the eyes are the mirror to the soul, see yourself for who you really are: a spirit being, a being of light here to have the human experience. Say "thank you" and "I love you" to your spirit for letting you have this experience. Now say "thank you" and "I love you" to your body for giving your spirit a home and a mode of transport in which to experience life on the physical plane. It may not be perfect; I will let you into a secret: none are! But it's your body and the only one you are going to get this time around. So thank it, say "I love you" and promise to look after it.

Our challenge to you is to do this for one month, 30 days, and then repeat the first exercise, step into your friend's body and look at yourself, write down what you see and feel.

"Old habits can't be thrown out the upstairs window. They have to be coaxed down the stairs one step at a time." - Mark Twain

Carpe Diem – Seize the day.

"We believe that we are hurt when we don't receive love. But that is not what hurts us. Our pain comes when we do not give

love. We were born to love. You might say that we are divinely created love spirits. We function most powerfully when we are giving love. The world has led us to believe that our well-being is dependent on other people loving us. But this is the kind of upside down thinking that has caused so many of our problems. The truth is that our well-being is dependent on our giving love. It is not about what comes back; it is about what goes out!" - Alan Cohen

> *"Choose a job you love, and you will never have to work a day in your life."*
>
> Confucius

2:43 Preparing to be a lomilomi giver

Principles for healing yourself and others:

Before you can connect to spirit and heal others, you have to prepare your mind and your body. For that you need:

Physical care:

- ◆ *Healthy, nourishing, life-enriching diet.*
- ◆ *Drink plenty of clean, fresh water.*
- ◆ *Regular exercise full of variety.*
- ◆ *Willingness to shift and create pono alignment with your environment.*
- ◆ *Make changes to improve your home.*
- ◆ *Experience different places and people.*
- ◆ *Willingness to speak your truth in relationships and set healthy boundaries.*

Emotional care:

- ◆ *Take time to commune with your core self.*
- ◆ *Find healthy avenues of self-expression for your emotions.*

◆ *Discover ways to recognize and release the emotions that build up inside.*

◆ *Be willing to let go of relationships that are not in alignment with your truth.*

◆ *Set healthy boundaries with clients, friends and family.*

Spiritual care:

◆ *Integrate a practice of connecting with your inner voice.*

◆ *Integrate a practice of meditation, visualization or quiet walks in nature.*

◆ *Listen! To all the messages that your dreams, life and nature offer you.*

◆ *Allow your intuition to guide you more and more acutely.*

Relationships:

◆ *Cultivate honesty and truth – pono clarity alignment – in all relationships.*

◆ *Honor those in your life – even if you don't agree with them.*

◆ *Find a place of forgiveness for all your relations and yourself.*

◆ *Set healthy boundaries and don't be afraid of losing a relationship – if it no longer serves your life, let it go.*

Clients:

◆ *Offer them aloha (acceptance) no matter how you feel about them.*

◆ *Set clear boundaries, physically and energetically.*

◆ *Hold your vibration! If a client comes in and they are down, don't allow yourself to lower your vibration. Invite them up to yours.*

◆ *Have a clear intention for the session.*

◆ *Clearing and cutting 'aka' cords (physical, emotional, energetic) after the session.*

Energy:

- ◆ *Energy is our life force and yet we act as if we have no control over it.*
- ◆ *Energy is the fuel of excellence.*
- ◆ *The higher your energy level, the better you feel.*
- ◆ *The better you feel, the more astounding your results will be.*
- ◆ *Our energy comes from our breath.*
- ◆ *Breath carries life and energy through the body.*
- ◆ *Engage in regular exercise, eat a healthy diet and get a good night's sleep.*
- ◆ *Be fully present and surrender to the wisdom of each moment.*
- ◆ *Live life with the spirit of aloha in your heart.*
- ◆ *This is the key to maximize the flow of energy.*

*"No act of kindness, however small,
is ever wasted."*

Aesop

2:44 Pule

Prayer belongs in lomilomi, it is our connection to divine light, universal energy, the spirit of aloha. Over time it has been transformed from traditional native prayer to Christian prayer, and recently once again transformed by modern understanding of energy and quantum physics into 'wilful, conscious intent.' Universal intention is the thermodynamic driving force.

It matters not what religion you follow or whether you follow a religion at all. What is important is that you consciously recognize and make a connection to the most powerful energy source in the universe, with the intention of channeling the energy for the benefit of another.

"Directed consciousness is the power that makes magic happen. Great focus brings great power. Every society on earth

prays, and what else is prayer but directed consciousness that sets up a link with the sacred?" - Rima A. Morrell

It's the switch that turns on the light.

"This transition does not diminish the authenticity of modern lomilomi; it merely demonstrates how the healing arts can change with times." - Robert Noah Calvert

First thing in the morning, count your blessings; a conscious state of gratitude creates a vibratory magnetic field around you that will serve to attract more blessings throughout the day.

At the start of the day it is important to connect to aloha spirit; this can be done when you first get up, at breakfast or on your way to work. If you forget don't fret, do it when you remember, but do it. It may just make your day unfold more positively.

Start of day affirmation:

◆ *Close your eyes, place your attention on your stomach and breathe in through your nose, keeping your attention on your stomach, switch your attention to your heart, breath out through your mouth with an audible Haaa – repeat three times:*

◆ *Say to yourself~ "What a beautiful (summer, winter, windy, rainy) day, may my eyes and heart be open to the day's lessons, gifts and blessings."*

◆ *And "May the spirit of aloha live in and radiate from me."*

◆ *Breathe in and out…*

◆ *It is done….*

◆ *Relax and receive, you have now called upon the spirit of aloha for help and healing.*

◆ *Mahalo and blessings…*

◆ *Breathe in and out, this time with a long sigh, type of… UUaaaaaaaaaaaa*

◆ *In your own good time, when you are ready, open your eyes… welcome to your day, you have connected to the spirit of aloha.*

Midday appreciation:

Take a moment's break, inside or outside it does not matter. Place your attention on your stomach and breathe in through your nose, keeping your attention on your stomach and breathe out through your mouth. Have a slow look around your surroundings and find something to focus on (it could be a flower, a blade of grass, a dog, or even the clouds) and for two minutes – no more – really focus on the item. If it's a blade of grass, see the colors, the sheen on one side of the leaf and the matt underside. Imagine touching it, really feel it in your fingers, smell it, and really appreciate its beauty. At the end of the two minutes, give thanks for the lesson, say "Mahalo" and go back to work. Practice daily, the eventual aim is to be able to feel the object's energy, its vibration, its life force.

Evening reflection:

- *The best time is just before going to sleep.*

- *Relax, clear the mind of clutter and take a few deep breaths, just as you would before meditation.*

- *Reflect over the day's events and find something that you are grateful for, and then give thanks. Find a lesson that you have learned, and then give thanks. Find something or someone that you felt blessed about, and then give thanks. You may not find all three in one day, but that's OK as long as you have one and give thanks with all your heart.*

- *If someone has wronged you or you have wronged someone else, real or perceived, surround the situation with love and light, forgive them and ask for forgiveness in return.*

- *Now think of something good you have done today, maybe something you are proud of, or a simple act of kindness, or a moment of love, of grace. Thank spirit with gratitude from your heart.*

- *Say "Mahalo and blessings" then go to sleep.*

Pre-treatment:

◆ *Here in this sacred space of love and blissful energy (breathe in)…*

◆ *I open myself to the power of the universe and the pure loving light of aloha.*

◆ *Please fill me with love, light and energy.*

Meditation:

◆ *Imagine a sphere of light (intensely bright, full of loving, healing energy).*

◆ *This light is part of the universal intelligence, the loving light of aloha, it will oscillate in a bright white light.*

◆ *Politely ask the sphere of radiating light to channel its light energy into your body for the healing and benefit of the receiver.*

◆ *With each 'in' breath your lungs will fill with the incoming light/energy of aloha and with each 'out' breath the energy/ light will fill your body, slowly filling every space, every cavity, every organ, every bone and every muscle until your whole being is filled and glowing with the vibrant energy of light.*

◆ *Now imagine the energy radiating from your fingers and toes, this now is time to start your treatment session.*

Final declaration before starting treatment:

◆ *I am full and radiant in the pure loving energy of aloha.*

◆ *I am protected by the light.*

   (Any negative energy will pass into the earth to be transmuted into positive healing energy.)

◆ *The spirit of aloha guides and graces my touch.*

◆ *With the blessing of spirit ~ let it begin.*

2:45 Lomilomi Healing Pule

E Aloha Mai
(Let there be Love)

E Mana Mai
(Let there be Power)

E Pono Mai
(Let there be Harmony)

E Ola No!
(Let there be Healing)

Amama ua noa
(So be it, It is Done)

"Always be kind, for everyone is fighting a hard battle."

Plato

2:46 Scanning the Body

Relax and center yourself. Take a few deep relaxing breaths. Stretch your fingers and your arms. Loosen your shoulders.

Sensitize your hands by rubbing them together for a few seconds. Stop, and then take another breath so that you are not just feeling the heat that you have just generated by the friction.

Begin to feel the energy between your own hands before you try to feel the energy of someone else.

Imagine where the edge of the person's aura is, then use your hands as an extension of your mind. It is important to scan for what is there, not what your mind might think is there. This is not a mental exercise, it's a feeling one. Start at the head and move your hands down one side of the body, keeping them in the aura, just above the body's surface.

When you reach the feet, move up the other side of the body, back towards the head. Make your movements graceful and keep your fingers moving as they follow the contours of the aura.

Make sure that you continue to breathe normally. If you hold your breath, it will keep you from feeling anything.

Keep your spine straight, or at least return often to a straight back position, so that you do not lose the nerve impulse and lessen your ability to feel.

Notice areas of the body that are cold or extremely hot. These are areas of imbalance and will need aloha 'oe.

Trust your intuition: the more you practice feeling energy with your hands, the more sensitive you will become.

> ## "Kind words do not cost much.
> ## Yet they accomplish much."
>
> Blaise Pascal

2:47 Creating Space

Creating space within the body is about removing blockages that deny the available space and restrict energy flow; these blockages can be of a physical or mental origin.

The earth's gravitational field is relentless in its efforts to bring the shoulder and pelvic girdles closer together. This compression has profound consequences for intervertebral discs, as well as the internal viscera. - Eric Dalton

A lack of self-worth makes one tighten and hold their breath. Most dis-ease is rooted in a lack of self-esteem. Many of us impose pressure on ourselves to do more and be better, and struggle to please others because we don't believe in our own worth. - Louise Hay

When you lie to yourself, your body shortens. Probably most of us have convinced ourselves we're not good enough (this is a lie) and have therefore shortened and tightened our core being. When we allow breath/circulation and feelings of self-worth to flow, we're on our way to health. When we find this freedom, or a part of it, we're able to help others find it.

Creating space is developing a safe environment for healing at wherever and whatever depth you want to go with it. That's why lomilomi has many levels.

> *"To cultivate kindness is a valuable part of life."*
>
> Samuel Johnson

2:48 Alo~Ha Breath

Hawaii's secret of paradise is aloha: 'the breath of love (Grace of Divinity) is in our presence'.

The real conduit of healing, the core, is in using breath as medicine. The Thymus is the switch and the Ha Breath the flow of energy that raises the vibration to a level for healing.

Gently talk to the receiver, ask them to be aware of the breath while lying on the table, and tell them to close their eyes.

Receiver:

◆ *Lie on the table, close your eyes, and listen to your breathing. Adjust your breath so you are comfortable with watching yourself breathe. Breathe in through your nose, hold it to the bottom of your lungs. Breathe out through your mouth with a strong HA. Keep your attention on the breath.*

Giver:

◆ *Pay attention to the breathing pattern of the receiver and try to synchronize your breathing with that of the receiver. When*

*you have gained synchronization, keep your focus on the
receiver but shift your breathing attention to your diaphragm.
Breathe deep powerful breaths beginning in the diaphragm,
at the solar plexus, the space between the lungs and the
stomach. If you are in rapport with the receiver, their
breathing will change to match yours.*

The Thymus

Next go to the Thymus Point which is on the centre of the
breastbone, about two inches down from the v-notch at your
collarbone. Place the fingers of one hand here, palm down, then
rhythmically tap them with the fingers of the other hand for about
half a minute using a few fingers – again, breathing in and out
slowly. The intention is to raise the vibration of the receiver to the
level of healing light.

The diaphragm, at the solar plexus, the space between the lungs and
the stomach, is the place where the power to heal comes through.
The diaphragm is like a drum, it is a vacuum. Breath inwards
activates the light energy; the breath begins and gathers power in
the diaphragm, echoes as it moves through the heart, then into
the throat where it becomes a healing chant HAAA! The outgoing
breath beats the diaphragm like a drum. This in turn raises the
vibration. - Harry Uhane Jim

*"Breath is timeless, as is the wind of time. Nothing is permanent,
thus providing the opportunity for change and adjustment."* -
Kahu Abraham Kawai'i

*Life isn't about trying to avoid the storms; it's
about learning to dance in the rain.*

Vivian Greene

2:49 Aloha 'oe

I have said it many times before but just in case you still don't get it, we are spirit beings, beings of light, beings of energy, embodied to have a physical experience.

We are at our very essence universal life force energy, energy from the source of life; as the source is divine energy, the ultimate level of 'love energy', then it stands to reason that we are also in essence part of 'love energy'. That is why we respond so really to love, whether it is given by a pet, a partner or channeled by a therapist.

The Hawaiians call energy mana and this type of love energy aloha, or the spirit of aloha; throughout this book I have referred to this type of energy simply as 'spirit'. I do realise, however, that for some the word spirit has religious connotations and for others, especially those with a western scientific background, it can mean some 'airy fairy' type of treatment.

The word spirit comes from the word spiritual and that in turn originates from the Latin *spiritus* meaning breath of life. Therefore the word spirit also means the breath of life energy from the Divine.

However, I do understand without judgement the group of people who have not yet graced this step on life's path.

So for future reference and clarity, when I talk about the act of channeling or simply engaging with healing energy, energy that is unconditional love, divine energy, the spirit of aloha, spirit, I will simply refer to it as aloha 'oe.

In many ancient cultures, the universe, the Divine, is represented by the symbol 'O' pronounced as in orange. Energy in Hawaiian is mana, in Japanese is ki, Chinese is chi, there are many choices of language. I have simply taken the first letter from the western word for energy and that is 'E'. Here the symbol 'e' is pronounced as in 'free'.

There are two ways of using aloha 'oe: the first and most simple is transmitting energy by placing your hands on the receiver. This level is not mind-directed energy, you simply shift to a harmonious state, a state of 'no-mind' thoughts just come and go, no attention is given to them, you open up to the divine moment of love and healing, the receiving of unconditional love. The transmitted energy then balances and harmonizes as and where it is most needed.

This is simple, but not easy, because most of us will, consciously or subconsciously, direct energy. The simple act of thinking about energy and/or thinking about the receiver will manifest a connection, and remember energy flows where attention goes.

The next level of using aloha 'oe is by way of wilful conscious intent. Here we request the presence of 'the light' then consciously direct the energy to the receiver with the intention of encouraging health and healing by the transmission of energy that balances and harmonizes as and where it is most needed.

The most important thing to remember is that you are not doing healing on someone. You are sharing a healing experience with someone, an experience where you both benefit to some degree or another.

Whichever method you use, the fundamental quality of the energy is love, and love energy does the healing. It is less dense than any other energy but is more powerful than you can imagine, it is even more powerful than you can **possibly** imagine.

It has a soft, yet powerful quality that can penetrate the stiffest muscle, the deepest recesses of a person's being or even those with the hardest hearts. We all respond to the presence of unconditional love.

Experience aloha 'oe with the following exercise:

Get a partner and sit facing each other, close enough to hold each other's hands comfortably. One will be the giver and the other will be the receiver.

All the receiver has to do is close their eyes and just relax and receive, without any expectations, be open to whatever you might experience.

Without touching each other, both of you should close your eyes, and just be aware of your partner's presence (two minutes).

The giver should now create a healing mindset, as though you were preparing for a session. At this point, remove any ego, don't force anything (five minutes).

Once you have achieved the right mindset, think of someone or something you love unconditionally. Find that feeling inside you and concentrate on it. You don't create unconditional love, just find the place inside where it already exists.

Now share this feeling with your partner 'the receiver' by gently directing the energy towards them. There is no force here, just simply focus on the feeling (five minutes).

Now reach forward and touch hands. Continue to focus on the unconditional love deep inside your soul and share this feeling with your partner. This time, imagine the feeling of unconditional love traveling down your arms into the hands of your partner. Again, don't force it, just imagine the feeling and it will happen automatically (five-ten minutes).

When you are both ready, breathe in through the nose and out through the mouth with a big Uuuuu (sigh-like noise); let go of each other's hands and open your eyes. You now may share the experience. - Kala H. Kos

"The ideas that have lighted my way have been kindness, beauty and truth."

Albert Einstein

2:50 Bone Washing

The finishing touches start with bone washing and the cleaning of the aura by pulling the old energy, emotions, aches and pains out through the extremities and throwing them away.

Thousands of years ago, healers identified the periosteum, the skin of the human bone, as the cache where memory of physical movement, memory of painful emotions, and memory of abuse lurks.

In bone washing, the giver places his or her fingers on the receiver's body and, moving the fingers between the muscles around the bones, directs energy to clear out the energy of the remembered wounds. Bone washing cleanses the fascia, and the muscle tissue.

Bone washing involves both deep breathing and visualization practice. If you can feel something then you can affect it, and remember energy flows where attention goes. So once you learn to feel inside the body to the bone then you can direct energy there for storage and healing/rejuvenation.

The bone washing modality can empower profound changes in the use of the body. Bone washing is done carefully, foregoing any pressure for focus.

Focus is best done with the receiver and the giver in thoughtful communication with the intent. Focus is the imagined idea of what to do. As the intent is to clean the blockages on the bone, the blocks will leave the area and become agreeable to intent of direction.

As the giver you will intend that the energy or base substance will stop being a logjam and flow on eventually out of the body.

You must be prepared that nobody leaves bone washing without a complete flow from head to toe.

"This is the medicine of the future." - Harry Uhane Jim

Bright rays of light would only shine

If each beaming ray should slowly combine

Such rays would create a path for you

A path in which you shall choose

Like burning sparkling flames of fire

Working together would fulfill your desire.

2:51 Laulima

Once the old energy has been removed, Laulima may be used to keep open the connection to the universal source of energy and the body's own energy circuitry systems, so that active energy can be transmitted and in a constant flow of cosmic waves.

This is a giving time; it's grace-receiving gratitude. Laulima is delicious. It's energy work in the least complicated form. It is not your energy at work, but the energy of spirit working through you. The touch with spiritual intention (aloha touch) can be quite miraculous. - **Harry Uhane Jim**

Often during this stage the receiver may be joyous and feel buoyant with energy. They may experience a 'starburst' moment, a feeling of infinite space, or a flash of sudden awareness, pure satori.

"The only thing worse than being blind
is having sight but no vision."

Helen Keller

2:52 Aka Energy Cords

It is important to keep a professional distance between the giver and the receiver. Therefore we would recommend that the aka cords that have developed during the treatment should be cut on completion of the session; by doing this you separate your energy waves from theirs. The method is very simple.

This is done in a loving act of gratitude, sending both thanks (Mahalo) and blessings to both spirit and receiver.

Place both hands on the shoulders of the receiver and thank both the receiver and the light for their part in the session. Slowly raise your hands above your head in the Kanku position, send love, gratitude and blessings down these cords, thanking them for their use during the session, wish them well as they go on their way. Separate your hands slowly, bring them down to your waist in a big circle while breathing in through your nose, lift those palms up to your chest, turn them over and breathe out through your mouth while pushing your palms back down to your waist.

Make a fist with both hands; with the thought 'until we meet again' sever the cords between the three of you by sharply and cleanly opening the hands and throwing any surplus energy into the earth for recycling. Now wash your hands.

> *"The difference between ordinary and extraordinary is that little extra."*
>
> Jimmy Johnson

2:53 Recommended ways to help yourself after a treatment session *(Advice given to the receiver)*

◆ *Rest for 20 minutes as soon as possible after treatment.*

◆ *Take it easy for 24 to 48 hours. Avoid doing anything strenuous such as housework or lifting.*

◆ *Don't engage in sporting activities such as golf, racquet or contact sports, or exercise classes until advised otherwise.*

◆ *Observe your posture when sitting, standing or driving – try to be as well balanced as possible.*

◆ *Drink plenty of water as this will help to clean toxins from your system.*

◆ *Keep a simple diet with plenty of fresh fruit and vegetables, and avoid alcohol, tea and coffee until your body has settled down.*

◆ *Avoid carrying heavy bags on one shoulder or arm as this will put a strain on your neck and back.*

How will you feel after a treatment session?

◆ *There is a whole range of sensations that you can experience after treatment. The most important thing to remember is that change is a sign that your body is beginning to adapt to the adjustments it has received.*

◆ *Feeling better: relief from pain as your body becomes better aligned can make you feel straighter, taller and altogether more balanced.*

◆ *Feeling worse before feeling better: while your body is adjusting to its new alignment, the shape and size of the painful area may change, or new pains and aches may emerge due to positional changes in your body. You may experience stiffness and soreness as the muscle tensions change and you may find previous aches and pains recur. These effects will disappear as your body settles down after treatment.*

◆ *Tiredness: you may feel tired after treatment, and may sleep well following the relaxation of deep tensions in your body.*

◆ *Headaches: the release of waste products as your body heals can cause headaches. Drinking plenty of water will help to flush them out.*

- ◆ *Menstrual cycle: periods may become heavier or lighter, less painful or shorter. Any changes usually settle once the body has adjusted to its new alignment.*

- ◆ *Dizziness: you may feel light-headed and dizzy due to the release of tension and increased blood flow to the brain.*

- ◆ *Medication: anyone taking medication, e.g. diabetics, will need to monitor their medication before and after treatment.*

- ◆ *You may experience reactions such as stiffness, tiredness, headaches, or even slight nausea. Rest assured, these are all normal responses to the treatment, and will soon pass as your body adjusts to its new alignment.* - McTimoney

Daily stretch/exercise (spiritual movement)

We normally associate relaxation with the stillness of sleep, trance, or meditation. But life is movement; relaxation-in-movement is the highest form of 'spiritual exercise'.

Slowing down in life, deliberately moving in very slow motion, amplifies awareness and expands time, enabling you to be conscious of every part of a movement or stretch – to notice and release any tension of which you would otherwise have remained unaware.

Have you ever observed a cat waking up in the morning? It will slowly and deliberately stretch and expand its body, separating each vertebra one by one. Each muscle and joint is embraced with gentle movement prior to any weight-bearing physical activity.

If the eyes had no tears
The soul would have no Rainbow...

2:54 Dance of the Butterfly

The Dance of the Butterfly is a beautiful way of connecting to nature, to get in touch with aloha and flutter between the physical and spiritual worlds. It is an experience in breathing, relaxation and connection.

Induction of the Butterfly

Stand with your eyes closed, feet about shoulder width apart. Raise your arms out to the side like a butterfly opening its wings and, at the same time, inhale through the mouth. Lower the arms and exhale, bending the knees and sinking down a little. Start fairly slowly and increase speed gradually to your maximum and keep this going for about two or three minutes. Then let the arms slowly relax, reduce speed of breathing and begin to dance, letting it take you where it will. It is good to tie a bandanna around your eyes and to dance in the dark, allowing yourself to go deep inside.

Dance of the Butterfly

Stand with your eyes closed, feet about shoulder width apart. Raise your arms out to the side like a butterfly opening its wings and, at the same time, focus on a white light above your head and inhale through the mouth. Shift your attention to below your feet, lower the arms and exhale, bending the knees and sinking down a little. After three breaths change the color to red and repeat three times, followed by orange, yellow then three breaths, then green, blue, indigo and then purple. Start fairly slowly and increase speed gradually to your maximum and keep this going for about two or three minutes. Then let the arms slowly relax, reduce speed of breathing and begin to dance, letting it take you where it will. It is good to tie a bandanna around your eyes and to dance in the dark, allowing yourself to go deep inside. - Kala. H. Kos

Catch your breath

Catch your breath, sit down in a quiet place, close your eyes, and take a few breaths. Breathe in very deeply through your nose until your abdomen goes out. Say the word alo to yourself or softly aloud. Remember, alo means to share. Then breathe out, softly saying the word ha, which means to breathe. Enjoy the moment and with your next breath say softly to your spirit self: "I share my breath of life with you."

Imagine that you are on a Polynesian beach just after you have awakened in the morning. Feel the warm, new-day breeze coming in shore. Smell the fresh tropical air, which always feels as if a gentle rain has just ended, and notice the subtle changing scents of all the fresh flowers misting around you. Feel your heartbeat and let it represent the deep drums of the Pacific gently thumping their healthy rhythm within you. See the rainbows that smile over the mountains on a fresh new Polynesian day.

Once you feel a little less Haole, or breathless, stand up and stretch. Remember just catching your breath is not enough to experience the full bliss of aloha. The true sense of aloha requires the catalyst of continually sharing the breath of life.

> *"It's very simple to be happy,*
> *But it's very difficult to be simple."*
>
> Rabindranath Tagore

2:55 A Smile

Everyone knows that smiling is infectious
You catch it like the flu

Someone smiled at me
And I started too

I looked around the room
And someone saw me grin

And when he smiled I realized
I'd passed it on to him

I've thought about my smile a lot
And realized all its worth

A single smile like mine or yours
Could travel around the earth

So if you feel a smile begin
Don't leave it undetected

Start an epidemic quick
And get the world infected!

A wave of aloha starts
With a single smile...

- Found at Heathrow, London

*"Remember that happiness is way
of travel, not a destination."*

Roy Goodman

2:56 Aloha Smile Technique

For a 30-second power trip of aloha that can restore and revitalize your energy, and connect you back to spirit, practice the aloha smile technique.

This is a deceptively simple yet quite profound technique that goes back thousands of years.

First you must get into a relaxed state, eyes closed and breathing deeply.

Find a point of calmness – waterfall, beach, and sun.

Feel confident, feel released, feel rested, and feel content.

Second, fire your 'happy' anchor without paying any attention to your thoughts.

◆ *Think of a person/animal/object that you love more than life itself, concentrate on this with intense focus for 30 seconds while touching the roof of your mouth with the tip of your tongue; at the same time connect the tip of your thumb with the first two fingers, do this with both hands.*

◆ *And know with complete certainty that you are loved back as deeply as you love. Really bring that loving feeling to a high intensity. (Sometimes tears will accompany the feeling.)*

Feel the heartbeat, the vibrating drumbeat of the body. Know that the tip of your tongue is connected to the sphenoid and in turn to the cerebral and spinous fluid that is the liquid soul of the body.

As the intensity wanes, remove your tongue from the roof of your mouth and open your hands. Breathe in deeply through your nose and focus on your stomach, now breathe out through your mouth, with a big Uuuuu (sigh sound) while focusing on your heart, smile to yourself and feel full of the joy of aloha.

Set aside half a minute every day for 30 days without missing one day, and repeat this exercise. After that time you will be able to experience the feeling of intense love just by touching the roof of your mouth with the tip of your tongue – a true aloha moment!

Discovering your mission puts you in a position of responsibility.

From this point on you must act as a torchbearer for others who still struggle with their spiritual identity.

Your life must be a testament that anyone can do as you have done.

2:57 Facing Future

Well, guys, a very big Mahalo for accompanying me on this nostalgic trip, revisiting some of the places of learning on my path up the mountain. Where are we and what's next?

I have shared with you some of my experiences; they are a reflection of my view at the time of writing, my interpretation of events and my conclusions. You may or may not agree with them, and that is OK. It does not make me right and you wrong or vice versa, we simply choose to see things differently depending on our world view and personal filters. Truth is the product of the mind alone.

Have you ever watched a game of football and then listened to the interpretations by both managers? You would have thought that they both had been at a different game. And that's before you add your observations.

The Hawaiians say that everything is understood by where the person stands on the mountain. The mountain, however, has many pathways and every pathway has a different view. A person knows and understands only what he sees from his own pathway. And as he moves, his view will change. Modern science now supports this multi-truth principle. As Buddha would say: "Don't always think that you are right." Expand your mind, challenge your existing belief system and change your world.

You can do this, as I did by studying Huna, shamanism, quantum physics and many other pathways. However, the way I hope you embrace is the one that you can start today, it's simply 'live a life filled with aloha'. Remember that aloha is love, love is magic and magic works.

My 40-plus year quest has resulted in this book, which is also an introduction to a beautiful bodycare system, a system that is underpinned by the principles of Huna and given life through the energy bloodline of aloha. As I now move into the twilight period of my present incarnation, it is my wish – no, my destiny – to share what I have gathered with the next generation.

To this end I have developed The Rainbow Course which teaches the Stardance™ techniques found in the Starlite® lomi bodycare system. The course is presented in a seven module format, each representing a color of the rainbow, and delivered in a workshop setting.

However, techniques without the magic are just techniques. Therefore, alongside the Rainbow Course we present the White Course. This course explores shamanism, the principles of Huna, mind expansion, and the 'aloha touch' – no one who has taken just one breath of the wisdom of light found in this course can ever be the same again. The White Course is not separate from the Rainbow Course; it is seamlessly integrated into the latter and allows a person to grow at their own pace. It is sponsored and supported by Azura and given free of charge to students, as an act of aloha~ in action.

In return we ask that you simply live a life of aloha and go MAD~ make a difference.

The bigger picture:

It is my wish that the Starlite® lomi bodycare system can inspire both academic and philanthropic actions, which as far as I am concerned are two sides of the same coin.

When students start the Rainbow Course they join our O'hana at Azura. Here they are encouraged, supported and inspired to go MAD, live and breathe aloha. Each little drop of aloha will fertilize the earth and encourage new young shoots. As the O'hana grows, the amount of aloha raining down upon the earth will increase, along with planetary spiritual awareness. Eventually, by natural progress we will have a cascade of aloha, a rainbow cascade!

I can't think of a better tribute to the ancestors of the oceanic people and guardians of the aloha spirit.

On an academic level I would like to see the Hawaiian people claim back their birthright. I would love to see a College of Hawaiian Healing Arts delivering a degree course to a new generation of professional bodywork therapists. Let lomilomi, Huna and the ancient wisdom of Hawaii claim its rightful place at the top of the mountain.

I would like to see the course cover such subjects as: shamanism; Huna; quantum physics; Hawaiian history; lomilomi massage; lomilomi bodycare; energy therapy; anatomy and physiology; physical therapy; injury rehabilitation and so on...

I don't see why this cannot be linked to the wish of Hawaiian elder Hale Makua's mother to establish a community school teaching traditional Hawaiian crafts and sharing their wisdom and knowledge, or a learning center such as the Keiki O Ka Aina. A student clinic could be established, open to the public, giving students much-needed practice, the community cheap treatments and the institution an additional income stream.

Students from all over the world could come and study, act as voluntary help to maintain and support the center, actually living aloha as they practice.

It has taken 45 years to complete my quest and develop the Starlite® lomi bodycare system, and I expect it will take another five to ten years to establish a worldwide network of practitioners.

It may be too much to ask to see the birth of a College of Hawaiian Healing Arts on this third rock from the sun, in this lifetime. However, as one great Hollywood actor said: "I'll be back!"

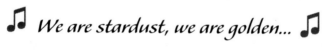

We are stardust, we are golden...

Joni Mitchell

2:58 Stardust...

"Imagine a pill more powerful than any known medication, imagine that the only side effect of this magic elixir is an euphoria hundreds of times more satisfying than that induced by any opiate yet free of the let downs and risk of drugs. Finally, imagine that this natural narcotic is completely free and that, when you take it daily, its effects automatically extend to those around you..." this is the magic of aloha." - Ramtha

I want to give you something, something truly magical that will change your life forever...

Remember – aloha is love and love from an oceanic point of view is not an all or nothing experience. Love can be used like grains of sugar. If you add a little sugar you can make things sweeter. The art is in applying the right amount in the right situation. If you add too much the experience may be overwhelming.

Each one of these words has a few grains or the 'essence of love' in them, some more than others: caring, kindness, affection, helpful, considerate, thoughtful, compassion, mercy, sympathy, liking, honest, and truthful.

Now here is a little trick, we are going to change the sugar for stardust. Now imagine a small black velvet pouch full with sparkling, magic stardust, just like in the Disney films.

Now here is the challenge when you find yourself in a situation where you can apply kindness, compassion, mercy, or any other expression of love. Imagine, really imagine, opening your little black bag, taking out the right amount of magical stardust and applying it to the situation, then personally taking the appropriate action. Remember, when sprinkling stardust you are actively engaging in the loving act of giving aloha.

The stardust comes from a never ending bag and will automatically multiply, but more than that, as you convert love energy into spiritual power through the act of giving, your life will become enriched and the light of life, your very essence, will glow in the stardust. The more you use it, the brighter it will glow with loving light – a reflection of your soul.

But beware! If you don't use it, the light will fade just like a dimmer switch turning down the lights in a room.

It is my wish that your light will shine brightly in the world.

♫ *Reach out and touch somebody's hand,*
Make this world a better place if you can ♫

Diana Ross

2:59 MAD

Are you living a life filled with aloha and have you grown enough spiritually to go... MAD?

I love this term conceived by Paul McGee (MAD) – it's about *Making a Difference* to the benefit of others. At Azura we call it 'Aloha~ in Action.'

In helping others we help ourselves. When we make a difference to others we also make a difference to ourselves.

Your story:

The question is what is your story going to be?

Start small, take a small step but in the right direction, take action today!

Do something where you are not the focus, but someone or something else is. The goal is not to broadcast how wonderful you are, but simply to offer your services or implement an idea that will help others.

If you Google 'volunteering' you will discover countless websites that can inspire you with ideas on how you can make a difference. A 10 per cent change can make a big difference, not only to others but to you also. You see, small actions over time can bring about big results.

> *"Anyone can dream, anyone can have ideas, lots of people do. But the value of dreams and ideas is when you turn them into actions. It's when you take the first step to make a difference."*
>
> *- Paul McGee*

 Love is magic and magic works...

Ripple effect

The ripple effect is a situation where, like the ever expanding ripples across water when an object is dropped into it, an effect from an initial state can be followed outwards incrementally

> *"The ripple effect is the notion that a single action has an effect over several different entities. When you drop a pebble in a pond, it creates a series of ripples that span out over the water to move surface plants around and disrupt the animals that may be on the water. In life, you need to understand how the ripple effect can affect you and those around you, your family, your friends, your business, and how the actions you take affect the people connected to you."* - Arnold Anderson

Inspiration:

One good idea and/or action can spawn several other ideas and/or actions that have been directly inspired by the first idea.

The gift from Azura

> *"Life on earth is dependent on the heat and light energy from the sun, the sun is our nearest star and starlight is the energy of life."* - Koko

The bodywork system is spelt as starlite, in order to differentiate it from Starlight – the children's foundation that it supports.

The Starlite® lomi bodycare system has been designed to dovetail perfectly into lomilomi massage therapy and is taught exclusively to lomilomi massage therapists. For they have already been bitten by the 'aloha bug' after hearing the 'call of the conch'. Anyone on the Starlite® Rainbow Course will automatically receive the gift of aloha from Azura in the form of the complementary White Course which contains insights into the magic of aloha. Azura do not request any payment for sharing the spirit of aloha, they feel that everyone is entitled to receive the 'grace of divinity' in the form of the aloha spirit without charge. They simply ask that the students as voluntary members of the O'hana pass forward 'a little bit of aloha' and touch the next person ready to receive its blessing.

> *"If we are to live aloha and receive the great pleasure, healing, and health it brings to everyone it touches, we must lead a much more kind, caring life. Only by giving to people and the planet can one find a blissful and balanced life."* - Paul Kaikena Pearsall

The aim of Azura is to inspire its members to go MAD, make a difference; it does not have to be one of the three core charities that are directly supported by Azura, nor does it have to be on a large or international scale. Look at your own community, look outside your immediate family, and ask yourself "What can I do to make a difference?"

Do some fundraising, help out at a soup kitchen, help an elderly neighbor, do their garden or wash their car, volunteer to help your local charity – even if it's just one day a year, it will make a difference.

Each year on 1st July (Azura day) we ask our members, the 'azurii', to donate the takings of just one massage treatment, to make a difference so that others may receive a little of what they have received.

The heart of Azura beats in West Sussex, a county in the UK. It's here where the office and training studio can be found nestled in the gardens at Snowhill. Here members of our O'hana run a cottage garden project for life-threatened children, and provide respite care for their families.

Our wish is that you go out into the world, live your life, have fun, and go MAD~ make a difference!

The O'hana based at Dove Cottage is committed to three core charities, but helps and supports many others. The three are The Starlight Children's Foundation, Morning Star and Chestnut Tree House.

Starlight Children's Foundation

Who we are

Starlight is a small children's charity which has a massive impact on the lives of seriously and terminally ill children and their families throughout the UK. We are the only children's charity delivering services into every children's ward in hospitals and hospices throughout England, Scotland, Wales, Northern Ireland, the Channel Islands and the Isle of Man. This year (2012) we will help over 500,000 ill children. We are there for these families in their time of need, lifting children's spirits in hospitals, making dreams come true, strengthening family bonds and creating happy memories for everyone to share and cherish, whatever the future holds. We know that happy children respond better to treatment and each year we help over half a million children to forget about being sick or stuck in hospital and simply have some fun.

What we do

Starlight brightens the lives of seriously and terminally ill children by granting them a once in a lifetime wish and also by providing fun, entertainment, laughter and distraction for children in every children's hospital ward and hospice throughout the United Kingdom. All Starlight's activities are aimed at distracting children from the pain, fear and isolation they can often feel as a result of their illnesses.

Together with healthcare professionals, we have developed a programme of year-round entertainment and distraction which helps over 500,000 children every year who are hospitalised for whatever reason. Sick children cheer, boo and hiss their way through **Starlight Pantomimes**, forget their pain and worry at **Starlight Parties**, play games and watch films on **Starlight Fun Centers**, take their minds off treatment with **Starlight Distraction Boxes**, and enjoy much-needed breaks from hospital on **Starlight Escapes**.

> *"Often treatment of cancer or other serious illnesses in children involves unpleasant and painful procedures; it is very difficult to make a child happy at this time. This is what Starlight does best in hospitals and hospices all over the country."*
> - Leading Consultant Children's Cancer Specialist

Starlight Wishes

If there is a seriously ill child in your care who needs something to look forward to, please put them forward for a Starlight Wish.

Starlight Parties

You can book a Starlight Party for your ward at any time of year. We'll provide goody bags, decorations and tableware, and funds for party expenses such as entertainers, face painters, disco, theater troupe and food.

Starlight Pantomimes

Twice a year, the Starlight Pantomime Production tours the UK visiting hospitals and hospices. Our pantomimes give sick children the chance to boo, hiss, cheer and shout – and forget about how unwell they feel.

Starlight Escapes

We can organize Escapes to suit children of different ages, with differing levels of mobility, indoors, outdoors – you name it. Be it a trip to the cinema, to the theater, a picnic in the park or one of our regular Escapes, we are here to help.

**Starlight is a charity registered in England and Wales.
Reg Charity No: 296058. Reg Company No: 2038895**

Starlight and Azura

Every Starlite® treatment, workshop or course supports the Starlight Children's Foundation through awareness and donations. The essence of the Starlite® lomi bodycare system is to share aloha with those less fortunate; we encourage all of our members, O'hana, therapists and clients to raise awareness of the Starlight charity and to regularly donate a percentage of their profits directly to Starlight via their website.

www.starlight.org.uk

Morning Star Children's Center

◆ *Was founded in Welkom South Africa on 1 January 2000 by Joan Adams; a second center opened on 9 October 2006 in Kutlwanong.*

◆ *"Morning Star Children's Center is a day care facility for underprivileged children who are infected with HIV/AIDS.*

It was born out of deep Christian compassion for the plight our nation finds itself in due to the escalating HIV/AIDS pandemic currently sweeping through our land. We are committed to restoring hope to the women and children of our region and making a meaningful change to as many families as possible. This we achieve through our optimum care, nutritious meals, appropriate medication, stimulating activities and the love we show to the 140 children attending our two centers. One aspect of Morning Star's focus lies in assisting our children's mothers/guardians become self-supportive by way of our job creation program.

We wish to share with you our trials and tribulations as we continue to serve the innocent victims of the harshest disease known to mankind and the neglected lives they lead."

"In 100 years' time nobody will care how much money you earned; but the world may be different because you were important in the life of a child." - Joan Adams - founder

Morning Star and Azura

Azura members were introduced to Morning Star by Linda Gardener, a good friend of ours. Over the last few years they have been involved in fundraising events and in particular the Christmas box appeal. Members, friends and family obtain a shoe box and fill it with gifts and essential items, such as toothbrush, knickers, and coloring pencils. The parcel is designated to one individual child at Morning Star and arrives in time for Christmas.

www.morningstar.org.za

Chestnut Tree House

Chestnut Tree House is a home away from home for sick children and their families. A place to spend quality time together, with our care staff on hand to help out when needed. So many new issues arise when a child develops a life-limiting illness — not just for the child but for their loved ones as well.

Our aim at Chestnut Tree House is to provide the care and support these families so desperately need, whether practical, physical or emotional.

Who we are

Chestnut Tree House is the only children's hospice in Sussex, England and cares for 280 children and young adults from Sussex and South East Hampshire from 0-25 years of age with progressive life-limiting conditions.

Completed in 2003, the hospice provides a 'home from home' environment with ten children's bedrooms plus eight family rooms, a wet and dry play area, computer and music rooms, a multi-sensory room and hydrotherapy pool. The house is set in beautiful gardens within an area of outstanding natural beauty.

There are potentially 1,000 families with life-limited children in Sussex. Chestnut Tree House offers support for the whole family, including psychological and bereavement support, end of life and short break care, and sibling support.

The hospice costs £2.5 million per year to run. Families are never charged for their care and less than 8p in every pound is funded by the government, so we rely heavily on the generosity, help and support of the people of Sussex.

What we do

Chestnut Tree House provides children's and young people's palliative care services. Children and young people with life limiting illness receive these services across Sussex and South East Hampshire.

The services we offer include:

♦ *Assessment, advice and information for children and young adults with life-limiting or life-threatening conditions 24 hours per day.*

- ◆ *Specialist short breaks, emergency and end of life care provided at Chestnut Tree House 24 hours per day.*
- ◆ *Specialist short breaks, emergency and end of life care in the child's own home 24 hours per day.*
- ◆ *Support for the entire family following diagnosis through the whole disease process by the multi-disciplinary team at Chestnut Tree House.*
- ◆ *Bereavement support which includes befriending, counseling and spiritual care.*
- ◆ *Support and advice on the transition from pediatric palliative care services to adult services.*

At Chestnut Tree House our goal has been to provide the best quality of life for children, young people and their families, and to offer a total package of practical, social and spiritual support throughout each child's life, however short it may be.

Chestnut Tree and Azura

Azura have been supporting Chestnut Tree House for a number of years, our members take part in fundraising activities including the annual Santa run (see our Facebook page)

www.chestnut-tree-house.org.uk

The Starfish Story

A young man is walking alongside the ocean and sees a beach on which thousands and thousands of starfish have been washed ashore. Further along he sees an old man, walking slowly and stooping often, picking up one starfish after another and tossing each one gently into the ocean.

"Why are you throwing starfish into the ocean?" he asks.

"Because the sun is up and the tide is going out and if I don't throw them further in they will die."

"But, old man, don't you realise there are miles and miles of beach and starfish all along it?! You can't possibly save them all, you can't even save one-tenth of them. In fact, even if you work all day, your efforts won't make a difference at all."

The old man listened calmly and then bent down to pick up another starfish and threw it into the sea.

"It has made a difference to that one." - Loren Eiseley

Now it's your turn, go MAD and 'make a difference'...

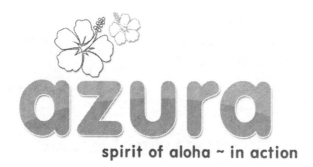

spirit of aloha ~ in action

Aloha ~ in Action

Our O'hana are a group of volunteers who wish to share the spirit of aloha with the world through the medium of complementary therapy.

The O'hana was started in 2010 by my wife Sandy and I, our immediate and extended family.

Our mission is to bring smiles and laughter into the lives of children who are terminally ill or who have a life-threatening or life-limiting condition.

The heart of Azura beats in West Sussex, UK where the office and training studio can be found nestled in the gardens at Snowhill. Here members of our O'hana run a cottage garden project for life-threatened children, and provide respite care for their families.

Azura also is the home of the beautiful Starlite® lomi bodycare system. All Starlite® courses, workshops and treatment sessions support the Starlight Children's Foundation.

This small charity entertains over half a million children every year in hospitals and hospices throughout the UK. They grant 'once in a lifetime wishes' to seriously and terminally ill children.

Anyone wishing to support this great cause, please visit the Starlight website and click on the donation page. Put in your details (you will be recognised for your generosity) and the amount you wish to donate. Please don't forget to put 'friend of Azura' in the comments section as when enough funds have been raised it will allow us some collective involvement.

Mahalo and blessings.

www.starlight.org.uk

In addition to our support for Starlight our O'hana have gone MAD and 'touched the world with aloha' raising funds directly for various other charities. For latest details please visit our website and 'like' us on Facebook.

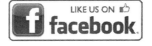

Bibliography

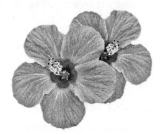

Agness, L. (2008). **Change your life with NLP.** Harlow: Prentice Hall Life.

'Ano'i, P. K. (2008). **Kamalamalama.** Honolulu: Ka'ano'i .

Arledge, H. U. (2007). **Wise Secrets of Aloha.** San Francisco: Weiser Books.

Borg, J. (2010). **Mind power.** Harlow: Prentice Hall Life.

Brinkley, D. (2008). **Secrets of the Light.** Harper One.

Britten, R. (2001). **Fearless Living.** Dutton.

Canfield, J. (2003). **Chicken Soup from the Soul of Hawaii.**
Deerfield Beach: Health Communications.

Chai, R. M. (2005). **Na Mo'olelo Lomilomi.** Honolulu: Bishop Museum.

Chang, B. (2006). **Riding Quantum Waves.** Big Bear: Destiny Technologies.

Chiles, W. (1995). **The Secrets & Mysteries of Hawaii.** Deerfield Beach:
Health Communications.

Choppa, D. (1989). **Quantum Healing.** Bantum Books.

Chown, M. (2001). **Quantum Theory cannot hurt you.** Washington DC:
Faber and Faber.

Cunningham, S. (2001). **Hawaiian magic & spirituality.** Minnesota:
Lewellyn Publications.

Dalton, E. (1998). **Myoskeletal Alignment Technique.**
Freedom of Pain Insitute.

Hall, M. (1997). **Practical Reiki.** London: Thorson.

Hamwee, J. (1999). **Zero Balancing touching the energy of bone.**
Berkeley: North Atlantic Books.

James, T. (1993). **Lost Secrets of Ancient Hawaiian Huna.**
Honolulu: Advanced Neuro Dynamics.

Kahalewai, N. S. (2000). **Hawaiian Lomilomi Big Island Massage.**
Mount View: Island Massage.

King, S. K. (1990). **Urban Shaman.** New York: Fireside.

King, S. K. (2008). **Huna Ancient Hawaiian Secrets for Modern Living.**
New York: Atria Books.

Knight, J. (1999). **Ramtha The White Book.** Washington: JZK Publishing.

Kos, K. H. (2000). **From Ecstasy to Success.**
White Rock: Gamma Group International.

Lipton, B. H. (2005). **The Biology of Belief.** London: Hat House.

Mackinnon, C. (2012). **Shamanism and Spirituality in Therapeutic
Practice.** London: Singing Dragon.

Melville, L. (1969). **Children of the Rainbow.** Wheaton: Quest.

Millman, D. (1995). **The Laws of Spirit.** Tiburon: H. J. Kramer.

Moondance, W. (2001). **Wolf Medicine.** New York: Sterling.

Morrell, R. A. (2005). **The Sacred Power of Huna.**
Vermont: Inner Traditions.

Namikoshi, T. (1981). **The Complete book of Shiatsu Therapy.**
Tokyo: Japan Publications.

Pearsall, P. (1996). **The Pleasure Prescription.** Alamda: Hunter House.

Provenzano, R. (2001). **A little Book of Aloha.** Honolulu: Mutual.

Roberts, L. (2008). **Shamanic Reiki.** Winchester: O Books.

Rutherford, L. (1996). **The Way of Shamanism.** London: Thorson.

Scully, N. (1991). **Power Animal Meditations.** Rochester. Vermont: Bear & Co.

Shapiro, D. (1996). **Your Body Speaks Your Mind.** London: Piatkus.

Stevens, J. (1988). **Secrets of Shamanism.** New York: Avon Books.

Suzuki, S. (1970). **Zen Mind, Beginners Mind.** New York: Weatherhill.

Vitale, J. (2007). **Zero Limits.** New Jersey: John Wiley & Son.

Weinman, R. A. (1988). **Your Hands can Heal.** London: Aquarian/Thorson.

Wesselman, H. (2003). **The Journey to the Sacred Garden.** Hay House.

Wesselman, H. (2011). **The Bowl of Light.** Boulder: Sounds True.

Williamson, M. (2003). **Everyday Grace.** Bantam Books.

Willis, K. (1990). **Tales of the High Rainbow.** Honolulu: Night Rainbow.

Willoya, W. (1962). **Warriors of the Rainbow.** Happy Camp: Naturegraph.

Wolf, F. A. (2005). **Dr. Quantum's little book of big ideas.** Needham: Moment

Testimonials

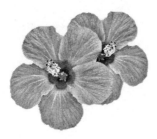

"Oh my goodness I love this book. I just couldn't put it down. I felt embraced with aloha from the first page to the last."

Claire Sommers, lomilomi massage therapist

"I love the fact that lomilomi is being presented as a holistic treatment and not just massage."

David Foster, Huna and lomilomi practitioner

"This has been a thoroughly enjoyable read; I've laughed out loud, cried a few tears and have been on a journey with the author. I feel like I had already begun my own personal journey similar to that described in this book before I even opened the first page, it has helped me find my own path and trust myself with the decisions I make in my own life."

Nataliee, event organiser and avid book reader

"Can't tell you how many times I have shed a tear.... of empathy, of understanding, of acceptance, of gratitude, and of sheer joy. This book has changed my whole outlook on life. I'm busy (& extremely happy) sharing my positive energy, giving more than I take and living my life to the fullest."

Sally Gurnham, Mother & possible future therapist

Discovering the sacred touch of aloha

Lightning Source UK Ltd.
Milton Keynes UK
UKOW031004180713

213994UK00011B/154/P